PARKINSONISM AND ITS
TREATMENT

CONTRIBUTORS

H. HOUSTON MERRITT, M.D.
Professor of Neurology, College of Physicians and Surgeons,
Columbia University

H. W. MAGOUN, PH.D.
Department of Anatomy, School of Medicine,
University of California

D. DENNY-BROWN, M.D.
J. Jackson Putnam Professor of Neurology,
Harvard Medical School

ABNER WOLF, M.D.
Professor of Neuropathology, College of Physicians and
Surgeons, Columbia University

LEWIS J. DOSHAY, M.D.
Department of Neurology, College of Physicians and
Surgeons, Columbia University

ADOLFO ZIER, M.D.
Research Fellow in Parkinsonism, College of Physicians and
Surgeons, Columbia University

WILLIAM BENHAM SNOW, M.D.
Professor of Physical Medicine, College of Physicians and
Surgeons, Columbia University

SAMUEL BROCK, M.D.
Professor of Neurology, College of Medicine,
New York University

EDWARD B. SCHLESINGER, M.D.
Assistant Professor, Neurosurgery, College of Physicians and
Surgeons, Columbia University

PARKINSONISM
AND ITS
TREATMENT

Edited by

LEWIS J. DOSHAY, M.D., M.A., PH.D.

Philadelphia   *London*   *Montreal*
J. B. LIPPINCOTT COMPANY

PREFACE

A GREAT need exists for a book on parkinsonism to which medical students and practicing physicians may turn for information. The writing of the book was especially prompted by the deep interest shown in this illness during recent years by general practitioners. The monograph is intended to serve as a handy medium for bringing the patients' problems and their management to the doctor, so that he may be better prepared to bring help and comfort to them. True, there is much that remains unknown with regard to the pathology, pharmacology, etiology and prevention of parkinsonism, but continued progress is being made in neurophysiologic, therapeutic and technologic research. Moreover, the future looks brighter for the patients, since the advent of synthetic drugs and the growing armamentarium available to the doctor.

I am deeply grateful to Dr. Denny-Brown for writing the chapter on Etiology for us; to Dr. Brock for the chapter on Psychotherapy; to Dr. Magoun for the chapter on Anatomy; to Dr. Wolf for the chapter on Pathology; to Dr. Schlesinger for the chapter on Surgical Therapy; to Dr. Snow for the chapter on Physical Therapy; and to Dr. Merritt for the Introduction and for valuable aid and guidance in the preparation of the text.

I am indebted to Dr. Paul F. A. Hoefer for assistance in the writing of the EMG data of Chapter 5 and for permission to use his photographs; also to the Association for Research in Nervous and Mental Disease for permission to reproduce photographs from Research Publications; to the Springer Publishing Company of Berlin for permission to reproduce their photographs in Chapter 4; to Mr. Kahoe of J. B. Lippincott Company, whose foresight and interest made the book possible; to Dr. Zier, my associate, for assistance in the preparation of the figures and material of Chapter 6; to Miss Elizabeth M. Fisher and Miss Virginia H. Fitzgerald for stenographic assistance; and to Dr. Adolph Elwyn and many others who helped with suggestions and advice.

L. J. D.

CONTENTS

viii   Contents

1

INTRODUCTION

H. HOUSTON MERRITT, M.D.

PARALYSIS agitans, or the shaking palsy, must have existed for many centuries before it was so clearly described by Parkinson in 1817. The condition is generally designated by the terms parkinsonism or Parkinson's disease. Either term is applicable. The symptom complex identified by Parkinson stems from a variety of causes.

There is no accurate information with regard to the incidence of the condition, but the number of afflicted individuals is large and there is no doubt that it is one of the major unsolved problems of neurology. All races are affected and there do not seem to be any economic or social factors of importance in relation to its incidence. Males are affected more often than females. The symptoms may develop in childhood as a sequel to *encephalitis lethargica* or as a manifestation of an heredodegenerative disease. In the majority of cases, however, the onset is in middle life or the early decades of late life.

The pathophysiology of the symptoms is by no means clear. All of the evidence indicates that the symptoms are related to a disturbance in the interaction between the phylogenically older extrapyramidal and the newer pyramidal motor systems. For the development of the characteristic symptoms, it is necessary that the corticospinal tract be relatively intact. The exact focus of the damage in the basal ganglia which is necessary to produce the symptoms is also not clear. Two facts, however, seem evident: (1) the symptom complex is most likely to appear when there is a mild diffuse damage to the basal ganglia; and (2) they are uncommon when there is a large circumscribed lesion in one portion of the basal nuclei. An additional peculiarity is that the symptoms may develop some months or years after damage to the basal ganglia by infection or other types of injury.

The etiology of the damage to the basal ganglia is known in only a small percentage of the cases which are seen at the present time. A large number of cases were seen in the years between 1920 and 1940 as the result of the great epidemic of *encephalitis lethargica* which swept over the world in the latter part of the second and the first part of the third decade of this century. In a few cases the symptoms can be directly related to intoxication with carbon monoxide, but any causal relationship between trauma, manganese and other poisoning is less clear. It is also possible that degeneration of the basal ganglia, as a result of arteriosclerosis, can produce the characteristic symptoms, but the pathological evidence for such a relationship is not unequivocal. In addition, there are few satisfactory criteria for the establishment of the clinical entity of arteriosclerotic parkinsonism. It seems most likely that the majority of the cases which are seen by the clinician of today are the result of damage to the basal ganglia of unknown cause (so-called idiopathic parkinsonism), and this may become manifest at a later age in some individuals than in others. Although the cause of the so-called idiopathic degeneration of the basal ganglia remains unknown, medical science is at present unwilling to accept the old concept of abiotrophy. It is quite conceivable that the degenerative changes will ultimately be found to be due to some intrinsic metabolic defect or to some exogenous toxin, such as has been suggested for the degenerative changes in the basal ganglia that occur in hepatolenticular degeneration.

The symptoms in patients with Parkinson's syndrome are strikingly uniform. The bizarre tics, oculogyric crises and dystonic movements, which were a feature of the post-encephalitic form of the syndrome, probably were the result of damage to parts of the central nervous system which are not usually affected in the common variety of the condition. The two outstanding features of the condition are muscular rigidity and tremor. Most of the symptoms presented by the patients can be directly traced to these two features of the disease. It is also worthy of note that despite the dramatic nature of the tremor in some cases, it is often less disabling to the patient than a severe degree of rigidity. Two striking characteristics of the symptoms of parkinsonism are their relationship to emotional tension and their disappearance in sleep. The latter fact, if more clearly understood, might give some clue to a more rational form of therapy.

Therapy of the symptoms is at best imperfect. Surgical procedures are directed toward an alteration in the existing disturbed relationship between the pyramidal and extrapyramidal systems. They appear to have some degree of success only when the corticospinal tracts are injured and a hemiplegia or mild hemiparesis is substituted for the tremor or rigidity.

The beneficial effects of medical therapy seem largely to be of subjective nature, since efforts thus far to objectively measure any reduction in rigidity or tremor have yielded negative results. There is no doubt, however, that the majority of the patients are benefited by the administration of drugs of the bella-donna group or the newer synthetic compounds, especially if combined with physiotherapy. It is likely that more efficient methods of therapy will be devised, but the main hope for the future lies in a discovery of the causation and prevention of the disease process.

2

ANATOMY

H. W. MAGOUN, PH.D.

IF ONE speaks generally of higher brain mechanisms influencing movement as the upper motor neuron collections, it immediately becomes necessary to distinguish between component pyramidal and extrapyramidal systems.

STRUCTURE OF THE EXTRAPYRAMIDAL SYSTEM

The pyramidal motor system takes origin from a restricted portion of the central cortex and passes by way of a long and compact path directly to spinal levels. A parallel but diffuse group of connections descending outside of the pyramidal tract, and hence called extrapyramidal, originates from several portions of the cerebral cortex and from the basal ganglia of the hemisphere as well and reaches the cord by way of relays, through the tegmentum and reticular formation of the brain stem.

Gross

The basal ganglia which contribute so extensively to this extrapyramidal system are cellular masses interposed between the cortex of the hemisphere and the cephalic portions of the brain stem. Their mass resembles a stout cone, lying on its side with the point directed medially toward the subthalamus and the base toward the insular cortex. The internal capsule, in its descent from the cortex, cuts broadly through the dorsal portion of this cone, separating the caudate nucleus on its medial border from the lenticular nucleus laterally.

The caudate nucleus is an elongate arched mass related throughout its extent to the lateral ventricle. The head protrudes into the anterior horn and the long tail extends along the dorsolateral border of the thalamus and, at its caudal limit, turns ventrally in the roof of the inferior ventricular horn to reach the amygdala.

The lenticular nucleus is buried within the hemisphere between the external capsule, separating it laterally from the claustrum and insula, and the internal capsule, separating it medially from the caudate nucleus and thalamus. A ventral sheet of fibers, the external medullary lamina, divides the lenticular nucleus into an outer and larger putamen and an inner and smaller globus pallidus. The latter is composed of external and internal divisions separated by an internal medullary lamina.

Microscopic

The caudate nucleus and putamen are continuous with one another anteriorly and ventrally. The similarity of their cellular make-up and to some extent of their connections, is a further indication that these two nuclear masses should be considered as a structural unit, the striatum, only adventitiously divided by the internal capsule. The striatum is composed of small and medium sized neurons, in a ratio of about 20 to one, only the latter giving rise to the myelinated striae for which the structure is named.

The globus pallidus by itself forms the pallidum. Its neurons are primarily of the large motor type with heavily myelinated fibers, whose white color in the fresh brain is responsible for the pallid appearance and name of this structure.

PHYSIOLOGY OF THE EXTRAPYRAMIDAL SYSTEM

Present knowledge of the fiber connections of the basal ganglia suggest that the striatum is primarily the receptive component, while outflows to other parts of the brain proceed from the pallidum.

A number of cortical strips on the convexity of the hemisphere and the cingulate region medially give rise to connections descending to the caudate nucleus, and a large part of the neuropil of this nucleus is of cortical derivation. Descending connections from the central region of the cortex pass to the putamen, and to a lesser extent to the globus pallidus, and some of these may be collaterals from fibers descending to lower neural levels. The striatum thus receives a large number of corticifugal paths.

One of the major subcortical connections of the basal ganglia is with the substantia nigra. Though formerly believed to be strio-nigral in direction, there is recent indication that many, if not all, of these fibers are ascending to the basal ganglia. The striatum also receives incoming connections from the center median and other diffusely projecting nuclei of the thalamus. Since these latter nuclei are the sites of

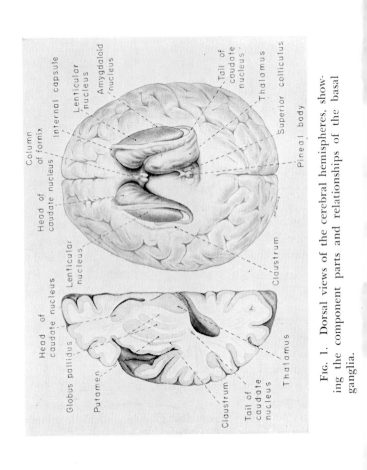

Fig. 1. Dorsal views of the cerebral hemispheres, showing the component parts and relationships of the basal ganglia.

ending of collateral afferent projections relayed by ascending reticular paths through the medial brain stem, the striatum can so be influenced indirectly by afferent messages from the periphery.

Efferent fibers arising in the caudate nucleus and putamen end entirely in the globus pallidus and all outgoing connections from the basal ganglia are, therefore, pallidal in origin. The external division of the globus pallidus gives rise to fibers which cross the internal capsule to end in the subthalamic nucleus, presumably for relay to lower extrapyramidal stations. Efferent fibers from the internal division of the globus pallidus swing medially beneath the internal capsule as the ansa and more caudally cross through it as the fasciculus lenticularis. These fibers converge in the subthalamus, from which a part of them pass to the ventromedial hypothalamic nucleus, while others are relayed to lower extrapyramidal stations. A large number of the fibers of this pallidal bundle turn dorsally into the thalamus, however, and terminate in the anterior or lateral part of the ventral thalamic nucleus.

The implications of these alternative sites of ending are not equivalent. The nucleus ventralis lateralis is known to receive the dentato-rubro-thalamic tract from the cerebellum and to project to the motor and premotor areas of the cerebral cortex. Connections of the globus pallidus with this nucleus have been proposed to be one link in a recurrent circuit from cortex to basal ganglia to thalamus and back to cortex, with focus upon the cortical motor area.

The nucleus ventralis anterior, on the other hand, has been identified as a major component of the diffuse thalamic projection system which is capable of widespread influences upon cortical activity. The im-

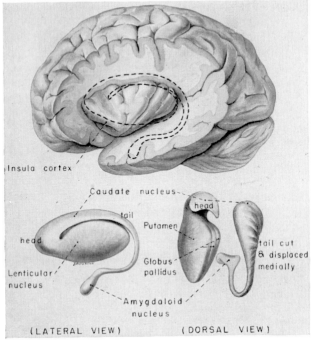

Insula cortex

Caudate nucleus

head

tail

Putamen

head

tail cut
& displaced
medially

Globus
pallidus

Lenticular
nucleus

Amygdaloid
nucleus

(LATERAL VIEW)   (DORSAL VIEW)

Fig. 2. Lateral view of the cerebral hemisphere with the position of the basal ganglia shown by dotted lines. Below are dissections of the basal ganglia in lateral and dorsal view.

portance of pallidal connections with this thalamic system is confirmed by recent physiological data. Such connections may similarly be part of a recurrent circuit to the cortex, but with widespread foci directed primarily to cortical associational areas.

Present knowledge of efferent connections from the basal ganglia thus indicate that their long recognized influences upon motor activity may be exerted both by descending extrapyramidal relays to lower motor outflows and by recurrent paths through the thalamus to the motor region of the cortex. Interconnections with the cingulate area of the cortex and with the hypothalamus provide channels by which the basal ganglia may influence emotional and visceral activities. Interconnections with associational areas of the cortex and with the diffusely projecting nuclei of the thalamus suggest that the basal ganglia may exert important influences on cerebral processes outside of the motor sphere and point to intriguing fields for future clinical and experimental investigation.

PATHOPHYSIOLOGY OF THE EXTRA-PYRAMIDAL SYSTEM

It is clear, from the many reports of lesions in the globus pallidus or substantia nigra of patients with Parkinson's disease, that injury to the basal ganglia is an important, if not the sole factor precipitating this disorder in man. It would be of great interest now to be able to account for the *patho-physiology of Parkinson's syndrome* in terms of loss or malfunction of influences normally exerted by the efferent connections of the ganglia just described. Large lesions in the basal ganglia of the monkey's brain have regularly failed to reproduce this syndrome, and it appeared that contributions to its understanding would not be forthcoming from animal study.

Recently, however, one of the most conspicuous features of Parkinson's disorder, an alternating tremor at rest, has been reproduced in the monkey by experimental injury to the brain. Different opinions exist as to the effective site of this lesion; one group holding that interruption of descending extrapyramidal paths in the midbrain is responsible, while another attributes the tremor to interference with outflows from the cerebellum. *The tremor itself appears definitely to be the counterpart of Parkinson's shaking in man.* Although slightly faster in rate, it appears at rest, alternates in antagonistic muscles, increases under emotional excitement, and disappears with voluntary movement, as well as during sleep or anesthesia.

The fact that this tremor follows lesions in the tegmentum of the cephalic brain stem and becomes augmented or disappears under conditions in which the activity of this part of the brain is respectively enhanced or diminished, as in emotional excitement or sleep, raises the possibility that it *results from an abnormal timing of descending extrapyramidal impulses* leading to synchronized firing of motor neurons in the cord. Appropriately timed excitation of descending extrapyramidal connections can be shown to synchronize the discharge of spinal motor neurons, and tremor-like movements have recently been produced by direct stimulation of the lower tegmentum of the monkey's brain stem.

For many years it has been reiterated that tremor and other symptoms which follow neural injury are not generated by the lesion, but reflect the abnormal activity of the remainder of the brain. This axiom has recently been extended by the proposal that, following injury to the basal ganglia or upper brain stem, extrapyramidal relays lying downstream of the lesion gradually develop a sensitization of denervation, rendering them abnormally susceptible to neural or humoral excitation from active neighboring structures. In favor of such a possibility is the fact that the drugs most

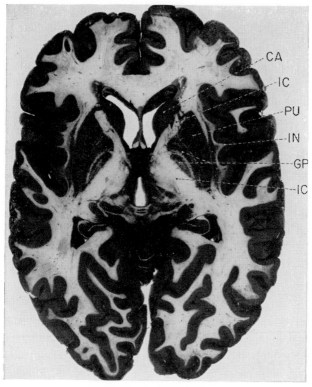

Fig. 3.*   Horizontal slice through the cerebral hemispheres showing basal ganglia. Nigrosin stain.

---

* Abbreviations for Figures 3 and 4 are as follows: AL—ansa lenticularis, BP—basis penunculi, CA—caudate nucleus, CC—corpus callosum, FL—fasciculus lenticularis, IC—internal capsule, IN—insular cortex, GP—globus pallidus, LV—lateral ventricle, OT—optic tract, PR—prerubral area, PU—putamen, SN—substantia nigra, SU—subthalamic nucleus, VL—nucleus ventralis lateralis of thalamus.

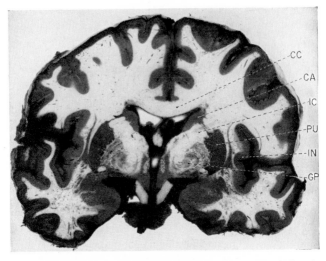

Fig. 4.*   Transverse slice through the cerebral hemi-spheres showing basal ganglia.   Nigrosin stain.

effective in relieving Parkinson's tremor in man have the common property of being anti-cholinergic.

Other symptoms of Parkinson's disease which may be reproduced in animals by injury to the cephalic brain stem are *hypokinesia* or slowness of movement. The effective lesions are most frequently located in the sub- and hypothalamus, or in the tegmentum of the midbrain.   Depending upon the extent of the injury, the animals may show *a loss of facial expression* and reduction of normal motor activity, or they may lose all capacity for movement other than reflex.   When *rigidity* accompanies this diminution of motility, it is of the plastic type, like that of catalepsy, rather than Parkinson's disease in man.

When, in animals with intact brains, stimulation of

these neural parts is tested against a background of existing motion, marked facilitation of movement results. Both reflexes and responses evoked from the motor area of the cortex may be augmented and the facilatory influence can be shown to be mediated by descending extrapyramidal paths which exert their effects at the level of lower motor outflows. It is reasonable to attribute the experimental findings and the hypokinesia of Parkinson's disease, in part, at least, to impairment of this extrapyramidal facilitatory influence.

3

ETIOLOGY

D. Denny-Brown, M.D.

PARKINSONISM is a symptom complex occurring in several distinct associations in such a way as to suggest that it has a variety of causes.

PATHOGENESIS OF PARKINSONISM

It is customary to list lethargic encephalitis, arteriosclerosis, trauma, syphilis, manganese intoxication, carbon monoxide, nitrous oxide and carbon disulfide poisoning as causes of *symptomatic parkinsonism,* and to classify the more classical syndrome occurring spontaneously after middle age as *"idiopathic" parkinsonism.* Yet, none of these factors satisfactorily explain the pathogenesis of parkinsonism. The most obvious and direct relationship, namely, that with lethargic encephalitis, a presumed virus disease, at once states our problem, for parkinsonism then may appear and progress at a time when encephalitis, in the usual meaning of the term, no longer exists, and when damage to the nervous tissue no longer shows any of the inflammatory process associated with the original illness. The relationship between any of the other factors mentioned and the associated parkinsonism is even more tenuous. The inconsistencies of supposed trau-

17

matic etiology are discussed by Mendel (1911), Patrick and Levy (1922), Wilson (1940) and others (Lhermitte, 1930; Alexander, 1941). Trauma and emotional shock profoundly disturb the ability of the known Parkinsonian patient to compensate for his disability. Therefore, trauma immediately preceding the first observed Parkinsonian symptoms is open to suspicion of the same effect in rendering latent symptoms obvious. A history of previous trauma to the first limb involved is not uncommon, but how could that induce a cerebral pathology? The onset of parkinsonism after a severe head injury is excessively rare. The occurrence of syphilitic signs and symptoms in association with parkinsonism is sufficiently infrequent to justify strong suspicion of coincidence of two chronic diseases.

The question of carbon monoxide poisoning is confused by several features, notably the rarity of parkinsonism as a sequel and the long delay (one to eight years) between exposure and the onset of symptoms. There is also special difficulty because the clinical disturbances are less clear-cut than in the spontaneous Parkinsonian syndrome. We have, for example, seen the immobility, loss of expression and slowing of motor response due to cortical changes following carbon monoxide poisoning called "parkinsonism." Manganese poisoning is reported to result in pseudobulbar phenomena, rigidity and a rapid tremor which more closely resembles Wilson's disease than parkinsonism. On the other hand, some forms of Wilson's disease may present a type of tremor and rigidity closely resembling post-encephalitic parkinsonism. The characteristic rigidity may also appear in a variety of other degenerative diseases when the process extends to the globus pallidus, for example in Huntington's chorea (Bielschowsky, 1922) and in progressive cerebellar atrophy (Mathieu, 1929). Further enquiry into these will only lead us further into the maze of extrapyramidal disorders of undetermined etiology.

From the various types of parkinsonism that have been mentioned, we may separate idiopathic parkinsonism (paralysis agitans), postencephalitic parkinsonism and arteriosclerotic parkinsonism for closer attention, for these form by far the greatest part of the problem. Idiopathic parkinsonism stands alone, not only by reason of its age incidence (onset most commonly in the fifth decade), but in its slow, steady evolution and uniform symptomatology (Denny-Brown, 1946). The infrequency of parkinsonism in young people before the epidemics of *encephalitis lethargica,* from 1918 to 1928, and the special clinical characteristics of postencephalitic parkinsonism would, for us, make it unlikely that idiopathic and arteriosclerotic parkinsonism are also the result of encephalitis, as suggested by Klaue (1940). Gowers (1910), for example, analyzing 236 cases of parkinsonism, found only two cases with onset before the age of 30, whereas from 1922 to 1930, cases with onset before the age of 30 were as common as after that age. Now the age of onset in fresh cases is again as late as in Gowers' time. Arteriosclerotic parkinsonism is later in onset, is rarely associated with the characteristic tremor, and is frequently contaminated with spastic pseudobulbar disorders.

The pathologic features of these different types of parkinsonism will be discussed in detail in the chapter by Dr. Wolf. With regard to the question of etiology, we may here note only that though circumscribed infarcts of the substantia nigra in the midbrain, result-

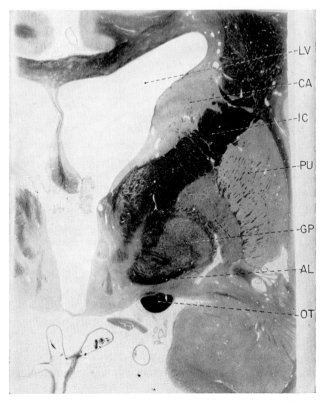

FIG. 5.* Serial transverse sections through the basal ganglia and brain stem (Figure 5 being the most cephalic). Weil stain.

* Abbreviations for Figures 5 to 8 are as follows: AL—ansa lenticularis, BP—basis penunculi, CA—caudate nucleus, CC—corpus callosum, FL—fasciculus lenticularis, IC—internal capsule, IN—insular cortex, GP—globus pallidus, LV—lateral ventricle, OT—optic tract, PR—prerubral area, PU—putamen, SN—substantia nigra, SU—subthalamic nucleus, VL—nucleus ventralis lateralis of thalamus.

ing from vascular disease, may occasionally reproduce the essential features of the rigidity and tremor; the characteristic combinations of the symptoms which occur in the diseases under discussion are produced only by *diffuse selective lesions*. Further, the striking preponderance of cellular damage in the substantia nigra found in postencephalitic parkinsonism contrasts with the variable proportion of cell loss in this situation, in the globus pallidus, and in the frontal cortex from case to case of other types of parkinsonism. This variation in anatomical location of cellular lesions probably indicates that the function which is disordered in parkinsonism utilizes all these extrapyramidal structures, and that variations in symptomatology represent disorders of this function at different levels. Certainly it can be maintained that the *more coarse and violent forms of tremor and rigidity* correlate with the presence of mesencephalic lesions, whereas the rigidity and tremor of frontal lobe disease are irregular and less intense. The proper understanding of the causation of these diseases is therefore a much wider question than can be answered by a list of lesions that affect the midbrain.

The intimate *nature of the cellular degeneration* has more direct bearing on the question of etiology. We have already mentioned the progression of postencephalitic parkinsonism in the absence of signs of inflammatory reaction or other evidence of continued virus encephalitis. Those who have been impressed by the long, latent interval in the appearance of parkinsonism in some cases of carbon monoxide poisoning propose that postencephalitic and idiopathic parkinsonism likewise represent a similar delay in the appearance of neural disequilibrium following encepha-

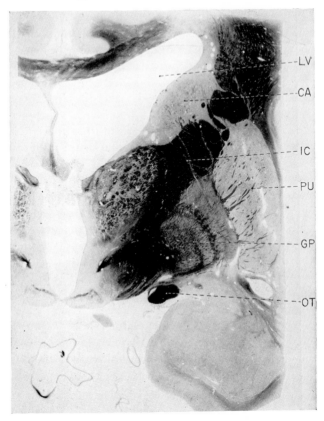

FIG. 6.* Serial transverse section through the basal ganglia and brain stem.   Weil stain.

litis (Alexander, 1941).   From this point of view the
continued presence of encephalitis is not necessary at
the time of appearance and progression of symptoms.
There are, however, some strong arguments against
this hypothesis.   Parkinsonism appeared during the
acute phase of lethargic encephalitis in many cases,

and in these, destruction of the cell masses of the mid-brain was already present (McAlpine, 1926). On the other hand, we have been unable to find any documented case of postencephalitis studied in the latent interval, with destruction of the substantia nigra that had not already led to parkinsonism.

An alternative explanation involves the presence of some type of cumulative metabolic disorder which ultimately destroys the cell. One such process is already known to neuropathology in the delayed response of neuronal tissue to radiation. Though this response tends to be massive and to involve cerebral white matter rather than cell bodies, it shows that *delayed mechanisms of neuronal damage* are possible. Another type of *known delayed cellular pathology is represented by Wilson's disease,* where the presence throughout life of a disorder in the metabolism of amino acids and copper leads ultimately to cumulative damage to the nervous system, and specially the basal ganglia (Denny-Brown, 1951). We have also learned from Wilson's disease that the same metabolic disorder can produce different accentuation of extrapyramidal and cortical signs according to its chronicity, intensity and degree of development. Though we have found no abnormality in amino acid or copper metabolism in post-encephalitic or idiopathic parkinsonism, there is a clear possibility that these result from some other cumulative disorder of cellular metabolism. Hadfield (1929) has maintained that siderosis (deposits of iron and calcium in the walls of blood vessels) of the basal ganglia predisposes to necrosis of the globus pallidus in carbon monoxide poisoning. The possibility that severe anoxia may in some way accelerate a cumulative

biochemical change of the kind that underlies siderosis and then have a delayed effect cannot be set aside.

POSTENCEPHALITIC PARKINSONISM

The cellular changes in surviving neurones in the
substantia nigra give no indication of the presence of
any histochemical change. Hallervorden (1933) has
reported the presence of Alzheimer's neurofibrillar
change in such cells. This phenomenon, which is a
striking feature of the form of presenile dementia
called Alzheimer's disease, can occur in less degree in
other conditions, notably in lipoidosis (Marinesco,
1924). Apart from suggesting progressive intracellular metabolic disorder, it is of unknown significance.
In postencephalitic parkinsonism this change is infrequent, and there is no clue to the essential nature of
the progressive process.

IDIOPATHIC PARKINSONISM (PARALYSIS AGITANS)

There is a more constant and striking change here.
Almost all who have studied this disease have been
struck by the accumulations of yellow lipoid, not only
in surviving nerve cells of the globus pallidus, but in
widely scattered areas of the extrapyramidal portions
of the nervous system, and in the thalamus and dentate
nuclei. *This lipoid* closely resembles that which is
normally present in some degree in any large nerve
cell, and which becomes more obvious late in life.
For this reason its significance is difficult to assess, but
its *unique prominence in idiopathic parkinsonism* is
commonly observed and is well illustrated in the beau-

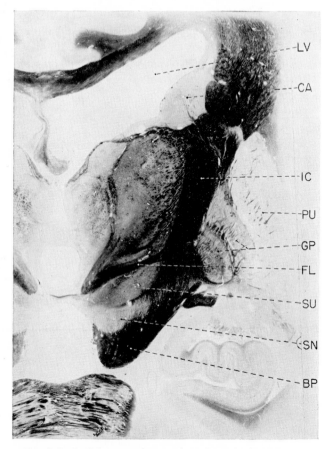

FIG. 7.*   Serial transverse section through the basal ganglia and brain stem.   Weil stain.

tiful monograph of Foix and Nicolesco (1925).   Bielschowsky (1922) has discussed the histological features of cellular damage associated with its presence in idiopathic parkinsonism.   The striking prominence of such a process as early as the fifth decade is at least one indication of *metabolic defect* of intracellular type, the significance of which should not be obscured by the fact that neuronal lipoidal inclusions of this type are to some lesser degree a feature of the *ageing process*.

Idiopathic parkinsonism has a well-defined hereditary liability, which has been estimated to be present in from 4 to 15 per cent in several large series of cases (Collins, 1899; Mendel, 1911; Wilson, 1950; Goslin, 1952). Kehrer (1930) collected records of 21 families with inheritance in more than one generation. Most commonly the affection has occurred in two siblings. Mjönes (1949) has recently presented a valuable personal survey of a series of 194 probands and 162 secondary cases belonging to 79 proband families, with careful statistical evaluation. This study yielded no statistical evidence of relationship between idiopathic parkinsonism and mental disease, ordinary epilepsy, psychopathy, oligophrenia or chorea minor. Some cases of arteriosclerotic parkinsonism with secondary cases were found, suggesting that this form of parkinsonism may also be inherited. Of special interest to the present writer is the report by Mjönes of the Lister family, a large family originally reported by Lundborg (1913) in his study of myoclonic epilepsy. Lundborg found 17 cases of myoclonic epilepsy in this family, and seven cases of idiopathic parkinsonism, and Kehrer (1930) proposed that there was some association between the two diseases. Mjönes reports that myoclonus epilepsy has now died out and that the family contains five further cases of idiopathic parkinsonism. In view of the fact that neuronal degeneration with lipoid inclusion bodies (most commonly of the juve-

nile type of amaurotic family idiocy) is the usual cause
of myoclonus epilepsy, and that extrapyramidal symptoms are a constant accompaniment of myoclonus epilepsy (Sjögren, 1931); this change in the Lister family
appears to us to have considerable significance. It is
strong support for a proposition that *cerebral lipoidosis,* becoming progressively modified in successive generations, may become the pathology of weakly hereditary idiopathic parkinsonism. The cortical disorder
which is so prominent in the infantile forms of lipoidosis becomes less and less developed, and the extrapyramidal disorder more prominent with later age of
onset. Such attenuation of a weak recessive gene in
successive generations is already known to occur in
muscular dystrophy, with change in type of the disease in successive generations. We have found a de-
scription of only two other families, one by Lundborg
(1913) and one by Berger (1882), where myoclonus epilepsy was associated with idiopathic parkinsonism in
parent and grandparent. Though such reports are
few, we nevertheless would regard these families as
important evidence towards a hypothesis that the familial, and by attenuation even perhaps the non-
familial type of idiopathic parkinsonism is a limited
form of cumulative metabolic neuronal lipoidosis. It
is therefore with special interest that we note that
Hassler (1937), in his careful histological study of
parkinsonism, found lightly staining metachromatic
cell inclusions in his Case 2, one of two brothers suffering from idiopathic parkinsonism. Hassler regards
these inclusions in his familial case, and the lipoid
in his non-familial cases, as non-specific histological
changes, but we do not believe that these cellular
changes can be so easily dismissed.

Most pathologists who have studied the pathology of idiopathic parkinsonism have emphasized the presence of lesions in the walls of very small blood vessels, and the corresponding small areas of rarefaction in the putamen and globus pallidus. The destruction of tissue is found in various stages which were called *état precriblé, état criblé,* and *status disintegrationis* by the Vogts (1920). We have been impressed by the absence of such changes in the brains of patients of middle age, which nevertheless exhibit the lipoidal changes mentioned above. We would maintain that the vascular disorder is more characteristic of the condition described below.

ARTERIOSCLEROTIC PARKINSONISM

This presents the result of diffuse affection of small blood vessels in the basal ganglia, and the globus pallidus in particular. Simple widening of perivascular spaces is a common and insignificant finding in atherosclerosis, but multiple small rarefactions of tissue (*état criblé*) is the more characteristic finding in "arteriosclerotic" parkinsonism, and *indicates a special predilection of the disease for very small blood vessels.* Such capillary lesions occur without occlusion of parent vessels, and it is therefore difficult to attribute them to arteriosclerosis as some have done (Alexander, 1941). *Their origin has remained obscure.* A mild variety of pericapillary rarefaction of tissue (*état precriblé*) limited to the outer segment of the putamen and caudate nucleus has been found in patients suffering from familial tremor by Hassler (1937). It is therefore of special interest that several families suffering from familial tremor are on record where one or more members developed parkinsonism (Kehrer, 1930).

Diabetes is seldom mentioned as a disease associated with parkinsonism by other writers. Patrick and Levy (1922) mention one diabetic in 146 cases of idiopathic parkinsonism. Mjönes (1949) and Kehrer (1930) record diabetes in some members, and parkinsonism in others in the same family. We have ourselves been impressed by the small but steady fraction of chronic diabetics who develop the symptoms of arteriosclerotic parkinsonism. Joslin and his associates (1952) in a recent survey of the neurological disorders in 913 chronic diabetics found 20 cases of parkinsonism. In very chronic diabetes a characteristic disease of capillary blood vessels in retina and kidney, in the nature of an intimal accumulation of "hyaline" material now identified as muco-polysaccharides, ultimately develops (Ashton, 1951; Friedenwald, 1950). This constitutes the Kimmelsteil-Wilson lesion in the capillaries of the kidney. These accumulations are not an index of severity of diabetes, and are thought to be the result of a metabolic defect associated with chronic hypoinsulinism, not necessarily of a degree sufficient to lead to glycosuria. These lesions are not found in the brains of diabetics without parkinsonism (Friedenwald, 1950). In the absence of any other known type of capillary lesions, this is a promising clue to the cause of the *état criblé* of arteriosclerotic parkinsonism with history of diabetes in the patient or his family. Only further investigation can show to what extent such a process underlies arteriosclerotic parkinsonism in general.

It is concluded that, though as yet there is no known certain single cause of parkinsonism, several considerations indicate that the etiology of the common

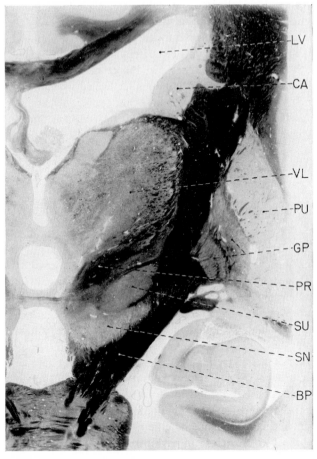

FIG. 8.*   Serial transverse section through the basal ganglia and brain stem.   Weil stain.

forms of the disease is to be sought in *chronic defect in metabolism*.   Pathologic studies indicate at least two different types of histochemical change associated with the common types of parkinsonism, and even in the postencephalitic type cumulative intrinsic neuronal metabolic defect is possible. The rapid advances in cytochemistry and in the knowledge of cerebral lipoproteins in the last ten years give promise that specific data may soon be obtained in relation to several aspects of this problem.

BIBLIOGRAPHY

1. Alexander, L.: The fundamental types of histopathologic changes encountered in cases of athetosis and paralysis agitans. Res. Publ. Ass. Nerv. Ment. Dis., 21:334, 1941.

2. Ashton, N.: Discussion on diabetic retinopathy. Proc. Royal Soc. Med. Lond., 44:747, 1951.

3. Berger: "Paralysis Agitans" in Eulenberg's Real-Encyclopädie der gesammten Heilkunde, Vol. X, 1882 (cited by Kehrer [16]).

4. Bielschowsky, M.: Weitere Bemerkungen zur normalen und pathologischen Histologie des striären Systems. J. Psychol. Neurol., 27:233, 1922.

5. Collins, J., and L. J. J. Muskens: A clinical study of twenty-four cases of paralysis agitans. New York J. Med., 70:41–46, 1899.

6. Denny-Brown, D.: Diseases of the basal ganglia and subthalamic nuclei, in Oxford System of Medicine, Ed. H. Christian, Vol. 6, Chapt. 11. Oxford Univ. Press, New York, 1946.

7. Denny-Brown, D., and H. Porter: The effect of BAL (2,3-dimercaptopropanol) on hepatolenticular degeneration (Wilson's disease). New England J. Med., 245:917–925, 1951.

8. Foix, Ch., and J. Nicolesco: Les noyaux gris centraux et la région mésencephalosous-optique, suivi d'un appendice sur l'anatomie pathologique de la maladie de Parkinson. Masson, Paris, 1925.

9. Friedenwald, J. S.: Diabetic retinopathy; fourth Francis J. Proctor lecture. Am. J. Ophth., 33:1187, 1950.

10. Gowers, W. R.: Paralysis agitans, in Allbutt and Rolleston's System of Medicine, 8:473, 1910.

11. Hadfield, G.: Siderosis of the globus pallidus: its relation to bilateral necrosis. J. Path. Bact., 32:135, 1929.

12. Hallervorden, J.: Zur Pathogenese des postenzephalitischen Parkinsonismus. Klin. Wschr., 1:692, 1933.

13. Hassler, R.: Zur Pathologie der Paralysis agitans und des postenzephalitischen Parkinsonismus. J. Psychol. Neurol., 48:387, 1937.

14. Hassler, R.: Zur pathologischen Anatomie des senilen und des parkinsonistischen Tremor. J. Psychol. Neurol., 49:193, 1937.

15. Joslin, E. P., H. F. Root, P. White, and A. Marble: The Treatment of Diabetes Mellitus, 9th ed., p. 469. Lea and Febiger, Philadelphia, 1952.

16. Kehrer, F.: Der Ursachenkreis des Parkinsonismus (Erblichkeit, Trauma, Syphilis). Arch. Psychiat., 91:187, 1930.

17. Klaue, R.: Parkinson'sche Krankheit (Paralysis Agitans) und postencephalitischer Parkinsonismus. Arch. Psychiat., 111:251, 1940.

18. Lhermitte, J., and Parturier: Syndrome Parkinsonian en apparence d'origin traumatique, en réalité postencéphalitique. Rev. neurol., 1:758, 1930.

19. Lundborg, H.: Medizinisch-biologische Familienforschungen innerhalb eines 2232 köpfigen Baurengeschlectes in Sweden (Provinz Blekinge). Fischer, Jena, 1913.

20. McAlpine, D.: The anatomico-pathological basis of the parkinsonian syndrome following epidemic encephalitis. Brain, 49:525, 1926.

21. Marinesco, G.: Contribution à l'étude anatomico-clinique et à la pathogénie de la forme tardive de l'idiotic amaurotique infantile. J. Psychol. Neurol., 31:213, 1924.

22. Mathieu, P., and I. Bertrand: Etudes anatomo-cliniques sur les atrophies cérébelleuses (Prix Charcot). Rev. neurol., 1:721, 1929.

23. Mendel, K.: Die Paralysis agitans. Karger, Berlin, 1911.

24. Mjönes, H.: Paralysis agitans: a clinical and genetic

study. Acta psych. et neurol., Supplementum No. 54, Munksgaard, Copenhagen, 1949.

25. Patrick, H. T., and D. M. Levy: Parkinson's disease, a clinical study of one hundred and forty-six cases. Arch. Neurol. & Psychiat., 7:711, 1922.

26. Sjögren, T.: Die juvenile amaurotische Idiotie. Hered-itas, 4:197, 1931.

27. Vogt, C. and O.: Zur Lehre der Erkrankungen des striären Systems. J. Psychol. Neurol., 25; Ergänzungs-heft, 3, 1920.

28. Wilson, S. A. K.: Neurology, Vol. 2. Arnold, London, 1940.

4

PATHOLOGY

Abner Wolf, M.D.

ANALYSIS OF THE PATHOLOGY

THERE ARE a number of obstacles to the clear delineation of the pathology of Parkinson's syndrome. One is the lack of unanimity as to the relationship of the various subforms of this condition and whether or not they can be related. Another is the lack of specificity of the cellular changes which makes it difficult to trace the extent of the disease process. Although it is now generally agreed that pathologic changes centered in the brain stem, in its broadest sense, underly the symptoms and signs of parkinsonism, the as yet incomplete knowledge of the extent and functions of the structures concerned with so called extrapyramidal functions furnishes a further hindrance to a thorough determination of the pathologic basis of parkinsonism.

In spite of these difficulties much information is already available. The pathologic changes in the central nervous system as they are at present known in the various forms of parkinsonism are as follows:

IDIOPATHIC PARKINSONISM
(PARALYSIS AGITANS)

As a rule the brain shows no obvious gross changes

in this condition. Rarely, atrophy of the basal ganglia
has been noted, associated with ventricular enlarge-
ment. Histologically, the findings have been compared
with those of *senility* (Lewy, 1913, Jakob, 1923), with
the emphasis transferred from the cerebral cortex to
the basal ganglia. The nerve cells of the globus pallidus, the putamen and the caudate nucleus undergo
degeneration. The globus pallidus was found by Lewy
(1912) to be more severely affected and this was confirmed by Lhermitte and Cornil (1921). McAlpine,
as quoted by Gamper (1936), made nerve cell counts
in the globus pallidus in eight cases of paralysis agitans
of Lhermitte and noted a 50 per cent reduction in
their number (Fig. 9). Lewy (1912) also observed a
great loss of the large nerve cells of the putamen, and
this was confirmed by Fünfgeld (1923). The predominant affection of the striatum and the pallidum was
confirmed by the Vogts (1920) and by Bielschowsky
(1920), but the latter reported an equal degeneration
of large and small nerve cells in the striatum.

The nerve cells of these nuclear masses undergo
pigmentary degeneration and atrophy. Their neuro-
fibrils are displaced irregularly and tend to coalesce
and clump irregularly. The nerve cell processes swell
and stain more readily and then become pallid, frag-
ment and disintegrate. The nucleus swells, the Nissl
substance disappears, and the cell body undergoes
dissolution. Satellitosis may occur about degenerating
nerve cells, and often there is a mild diffuse astrocytosis with a modest increase in glial fibers. Lipoid glob-
ules and pigment granules are seen in the cytoplasm
of some of the reactive glia, predominantly the microglia. Adjacent to degenerating neurons and along their
disintegrating processes, basophilic bodies, the size of

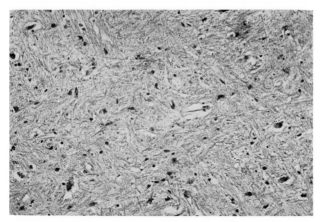

Fig. 9.   Idiopathic parkinsonism. Man, 63 years of age. Diminution of nerve cells in globus pallidus. Pigmentary atrophy of remaining nerve cells. Hematoxylin-eosin stain. (× 170)

glial nuclei, are encountered. These often coalesce into mulberrylike masses and are found to contain iron salts, and albuminoid and lipid material (Fig. 10). They are also encountered in the walls of local blood vessels and in their perivascular spaces. This has been interpreted as being simply an intermediate or end product of degeneration of parenchymal elements in an area notably rich in iron and not specific for parkinsonism. In many instances no abnormal changes are observed in myelin stains.

Jelgersma (1908) noted pallor and a reduction in volume of the ansa lenticularis (Fig. 11), and this was confirmed by Foix and Nicolesco (1923). Similar changes were recorded in the fasciculus lenticularis, the zona incerta and the capsule of the corpus Luysi. Both coarse and fine fibers may be irregularly dimin-

38   Pathology

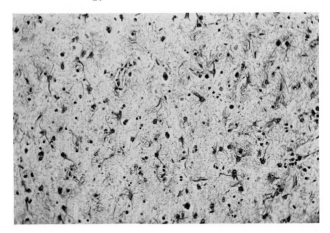

Fig. 10.   Idiopathic parkinsonism. Man, 63 years of age.
Disappearance of all large nerve cells and most of the small
nerve cells in the putamen. The remaining small nerve cells
are atrophic and there is a diffuse astrocytosis. Hematoxylin-
eosin stain. (× 170)

ished in number in the striatum and the pallidum.
The Vogts noted a perivascular rarefaction and dis-
integration of the neural tissue of the striatum and
the pallidum leading to a lacunar or cribriform appearance of the parenchyma. This perivascular degeneration was described as involving both neurons and
myelin sheaths. Bielchowsky (1922) confirmed the ob-
servations of the Vogts and attributed the lesions to
a capillary fibrosis. This conception of the Vogts and
of Bielschowsky of a *vascular basis for the tissue degeneration* is in sharp contrast with that of Lewy
(1913), Jakob (1923) and Lhermitte and Cornil (1921),
who regarded the pathologic process in idiopathic parkinsonism as akin to that of *senility, occurring in the
presenile period.*

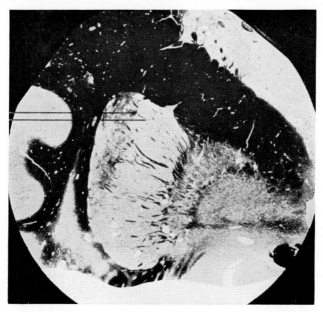

Fig. 11. Idiopathic parkinsonism. Woman, 68 years of age. Degeneration of the ansa lenticularis and the lenticular and thalamic fasciculi. Pallor of pallidum and reduction of fibers in putamen. Myelin stain. (F. H. Lewy: Die Lehre vom Tonus und der Bewegung, 1923, p. 214)

Some have found the substantia nigra to be the structure predominantly involved in idiopathic parkinsonism. Tretiakoff (1919), Foix and Nicolesco (1923) and Davison (1942) always found this structure to be most severely affected in idiopathic parkinsonism. However, the Vogts (1920), Neustaedter and Liber (1937) and Denny-Brown (1946) regarded the changes in this structure as relatively insignificant. The last declared that he was not convinced that the

substantia nigra is ever wholly unaffected in true idiopathic parkinsonism.

A series of additional structures in the brain have
been cited as being concomitantly affected in idiopathic parkinsonism. These include the basal, tube-
ral, paraventricular and occasionally other hypothalamic nuclei; the parasympathetic oculomotor, trigem-
inal and dorsal vagus nuclei and less often the inferior
olives, the red nucleus and zona incerta.

Although a great deal of disagreement exists as to
particulars, at present it is generally agreed that the
principal pathologic changes in idiopathic parkinsonism are confined to, or center about, the globus pallidus, the putamen, the caudate nucleus and the substantia nigra. Most of the authorities attribute the
predominant features of the disease to changes in the
globus pallidus and in the large cells of the putamen
and the caudate nucleus, while fewer insist on the
constant or even principal changes in the substantia
nigra. The histologic character of the degenerative
changes in the nerve cells and the reaction to these
most nearly approximate those seen in senility, but
occur in the presenile period and in the basal ganglia,
rather than in the cortex. Most agree that vascular
changes have no pathogenic significance.

POSTENCEPHALITIC PARKINSONISM

This sequel of epidemic encephalitis (lethargic, or
Von Economo's encephalitis) may supervene at an
interval of from days to decades following the initial
acute disease process. The majority of those who have
investigated this condition hold that its prime feature
is a patholigic change in the substantia nigra (Gold-

stein, 1922; Spatz, 1924; Jakob, 1923, etc.), while involvement of other structures is less prominent and rarely denied.

Grossly, the substantia nigra is found to be reduced in size and pallid (Figs. 12 and 13). Histologically, there is a reduction in the number of nigral nerve cells, which Davison (1942) estimated to be a diminution to one tenth the normal number (Fig. 14). This is seen in the zona compacta and to a lesser degree in the zona reticulata. Surviving nerve cells are often shrunken, and some are pallid. Their nuclei may be deeply staining and distorted. Melanin remaining from destroyed nerve cells persists as coarse granules free in the tissue or in hypertrophied microglia, some of which are rounded off and in perivascular spaces. There is a relative increase in glial elements due to the glial reaction and to the concentration of such cells. In instances where parkinsonism has developed shortly after the acute disease, microglial proliferation may be lively, focal and productive of elongated, rod-like elements. Perivascular lymphocytic infiltration is present in the substantia nigra in such instances and has been described as persisting for years following the initial disease. Some have interpreted this as evidence of a persistence of a viral infection. This remains in doubt, since it cannot be confirmed by the direct demonstration of such virus in the postencephalitic state, none having been demonstrated in the primary condition, and because of the frequent observation of nonspecific perivascular lymphocytic infiltration in the brain stem of apparently normal individuals.

Degeneration of nerve cells and their fibers has been described in other structures, notably in the globus

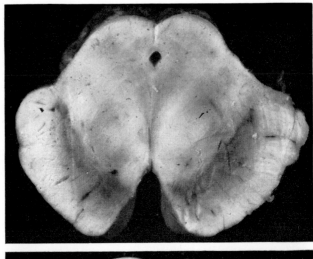

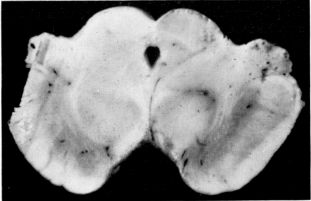

FIG. 12 (*Top*).   Normal midbrain.
FIG. 13 (*Bottom*).   Postencephalitic parkinsonism. Degeneration of substantia nigra.

pallidus (Secretan and Hedinger, 1922), the putamen and the caudate nuclei (Urechia, 1922), the locus caer-

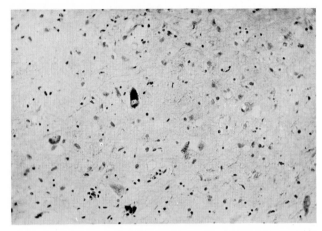

Fig. 14. Postencephalitic parkinsonism. Man, 58 years of age. Marked loss of nerve cells in substantia nigra. Hematoxylin-eosin stain. (× 170)

uleus, the basal nucleus, the hypothalamic nuclei, the dentate nuclei, the inferior olives, etc.

In assessing the pathologic findings to the clinical phenomena, there is no doubt, as attested to by one's own cases, of the importance of the regular and severe changes in the substantia nigra. In view of the distribution of lesions in the acute stage of epidemic encephalitis, the possibility of the subsequent appearance of degenerative changes in other structures, referred to above, cannot be denied. However, they are often difficult to demonstrate.

"ARTERIOSCLEROTIC PARKINSONISM"

Some instances of parkinsonism have been classified as arteriosclerotic. This has been based largely on the appearance of the Parkinsonian syndrome in individuals with cerebral arteriosclerosis who have had areas of softening or diffuse degeneration in the basal ganglia. However, the frequency of infarcts in the basal ganglia in the presence of arteriosclerosis, cf arteriosclerosis coincident with hypertension, of hypertension, and of circulatory disturbances in other diseases is so great that the strikingly smaller incidence of parkinsonism is disturbing in this connection.

When parkinsonism has been described in the presence of arteriosclerosis, rigidity has been its chief feature, with little or no tremor. Marie (1901) attributed the extrapyramidal syndrome to so-called lacunar lesions in the brain. Foerster (1909), describing similar cases as arteriosclerotic muscle rigidity, referred the clinical findings to small focal lesions in the ponto-cerebellar pathways. Lhermitte (1922) recorded similar cases as examples of a *syndrom strié d'origine lacunaire*. Jakob (1923) reported loculation of the basal ganglia in this condition and less commonly microscopic lesions. Critchley (1929) reviewed the subject and set up a number of clinical subvarieties. Keschner and Sloane (1931) reported on cases of arteriosclerotic parkinsonism and confessed that in some instances it was difficult to distinguish between the pathologic changes in idiopathic and arteriosclerotic parkinsonism.

Davison (1942) recorded 18 cases of arteriosclerotic parkinsonism. Acute and chronic degenerative changes in neurons and focal areas of dissolution with phagocyte formation were widely disseminated in the central nervous system. The structures most consistently and severely involved and *always bilaterally* were the globus pallidus and the substantia nigra, the latter slightly less than the former. The corpus striatum and the thalamus also showed changes, but these were less extensive. The globus pallidus often had a lacunar appearance, and there was shrinkage of the ansa lenticularis. Myelin sheaths and axons in the globus pallidus were more severely degenerated than in Davison's cases of idiopathic and postencephalitic parkinsonism. Fewer and milder changes of a like nature were seen in the red nucleus and the locus coeruleus. Areas 4, 6 and 8 of the cerebral cortex showed pathologic changes in all but four cases. Arteriosclerotic changes were present in vessels of the affected areas, in particular in the globus pallidus, where calcification was described as striking. All but one of Davison's cases were over 50, and 11 were over 60, a proper age for arteriosclerosis.

Denny-Brown (1946), in summarizing the pathology of arteriosclerotic parkinsonism, describes diffusely distributed small lacunae or foci of softening in the external capsule, the corpus striatum and the globus pallidus. These are golden yellow in color and vary in size from 1 to 3 mm. A marked loss of nerve cells in the corpus striatum and the globus pallidus is attended by considerable glial proliferation. Denny-Brown interprets the iron pigment in the older lesions as evidence that they were primarily hemorrhagic. He records arteriosclerosis in the vessels of the basal ganglia but discounts calcification in their walls as a common phenomenon after middle life. The substantia nigra is similarly but less constantly affected. Lacunar lesions may be widely disseminated in the cerebral cortex and white matter.

Syphilitic Parkinsonism

Autopsied cases in which syphilis was considered

to be of etiologic significance have been reported by
Mella and Katz (1924), Nonne (1924) and others.
However, the association of neurosyphilis and parkinsonism is probably fortuitous in these cases. The
likely concidence of two independent conditions is
perhaps most obvious in cases of long-standing tabes
dorsalis in which parkinsonism has supervened late in
the course of the first disease.

Intoxication and Parkinsonism

Carbon Monxide Poisoning. In an individual who
suffers acute poisoning of this type and does not suc-
cumb, as is usually the case, parkinsonism may develop
among other symptoms and signs within several
months to five years and remain stationary thereafter.
Many pathologic reports (Wohlwill, 1921; Grinker,
1925; Alexander, 1942) have clearly established the
bilateral necrosis of the anterior portion of the globus
pallidus, which is the most characteristic lesion in this
form of intoxication. The lesions resemble those that
result from a circulatory disturbance, and among the
acute changes in the neurones is ischemic necrosis.
This proceeds to total dissolution of all elements in
the involved area, with extensive phagocyte formation.
In the stage in which parkinsonism has appeared,
roughly symmetrical cysts are seen grossly in the anterior portion of each globus pallidus and are indis-
tinguishable from the result of infarcts in the same
areas. The predilection of the process for the globus
pallidus has been attributed by Hiller (1924) and
Spielmeyer (1925) to a combination of localized differ-
ence in the capillary network and vasoparalysis.

That the characteristic localization of the lesions is
not due to a special susceptibility of the globus pal-

lidus to carbon monoxide seems likely for a number of reasons. Much of the globus pallidus is unaffected; other portions of the brain such as the cerebral cortex, the cerebral white matter, the cerebellum and the substantia nigra are often involved; and other toxins such as nitrous oxide (Courville, 1939), manganese (Grinker, 1925), carbon disulfide (Negro, 1930) and phosphorus (Stiefler, 1923) may rarely lead to degeneration of the globus pallidus and in some instances to a Parkinsonian syndrome.

REFERENCES

Alexander, L.: The fundamental types of histopathological changes encountered in cases of athetosis and paralysis agitans, *in* Diseases of the Basal Ganglia, A. Res. Nerv. & Ment. Dis., Proc. **21**:334, 1942.

Bielschowsky, M.: Einige Bemerkungen zur normalen und pathologischen Histologie des Schweif- und Linsenkerns, J. Psychol. u. Neurol. **25**:1, 1920.

————: Weitere Bemerkungen zur normalen und pathologischen Histologie des striaren Systems, J. Psychol. u. Neurol. **27**:233, 1922.

Courville, C. B.: Untoward Effects of Nitrous Oxide Anesthesia, Mountain View, Cal., Pacific Press, 1939.

Critchley, M.: Arteriosclerotic parkinsonism, Brain **52**:23, 1929.

Davison, C.: The role of the globus pallidus and substantia nigra in the production of rigidity and tremor. A clinico-pathologic study of paralysis agitans, *in* Diseases of the Basal Ganglia, A. Res. Nerv. & Ment. Dis., Proc. **21**:267, 1942.

Denny-Brown, D.: Diseases of the Basal Ganglia and Subthalamic Nuclei, New York, Oxford, 1946.

Foerster, O.: Die arteriosclerotische Muskelstarre, Allg. Ztschr. d. Psychiat. **66**:902, 1909.

Foix, C.: Les lésions anatomiques de la maladie de Parkinson, Rev. neurol. **28**:593, 1921.

Foix, C., and Nicolesco, J.: Sur les connexions du locus niger de Soemmering, Encéphale 18:553, 1923.

Fünfgeld, E.: Zur pathologischen Anatomie der paralysis agitans, Ztschr. d. ges. Neurol. u. Psychiat. 81:187, 1923.

Gamper, E.: Paralysis agitans, in Bumke, O., and Foerster, O.: Handb. d. Neurol. 16:757, Berlin, Julius Springer, 1936.

Goldstein, K.: Über anatomische Veränderungen (Atrophie der Substantia nigra) bei postencephalitischem Parkinsonismus, Ztschr. d. ges. Neurol. u. Psychiat. 76:627, 1922.

Grinker, R. R.: Über ein Fall von Leuchtgasvergiftung mit doppelseitiger Pallidumerweichung, Ztschr. d. ges. Neurol. u. Psychiat. 98:443, 1925.

Jakob, A.: Die extrapyramidalen Erkrankungen, Monogr. a. d. Gesamtgeb. d. Neurol. u. Psychiat., Berlin, Julius Springer, 1923.

Jelgersma, G.: Neue anatomischen Befunde bei Paralysis agitans und bei chronischer Chorea, Zentralbl. Neurol. 27:995, 1908.

Keschner, M., and Sloane, P.: Encephalitic, idiopathic and arteriosclerotic parkinsonism, Arch. Neurol. & Psychiat. 25:1011, 1931.

Lewy, F. H.: Die Lehre vom Tonus und der Bewegung, Monogr. a. d. Gesamtgeb. d. Neurol. u. Psychiat., Berlin, Julius Springer, 1923.

————: Die pathologische Anatomie der Paralysis agitans, Lewandowsky's Handb. 3:920, 1912.

————: Zur pathologischen Anatomie der Paralysis agitans, Deutsche Ztschr. Nerven. 50:50, 1913.

Lhermitte, J.: Les syndromes anatomo-cliniques du corps strié, chez le vieillard, Rev. neurol. 29:406, 1922.

Lhermitte, J., and Cornil, L.: Un cas de syndrome parkinsonien: Lacunes symétriques dans les globus pallidus; Rev. neurol. 28:189, 1921.

————: Recherches anatomiques sur la maladie de parkinson, Rev. neurol. 37:587, 1921.

Marie, P.: Foyers lacunaires de désintégration et différents autres états cavitaires du cerveau, Rev. méd. 21:281, 1901.

Mella, H., and Katz, S. E.: Neurosyphilis as an etiological

factor in the parkinsonian syndrome, J. Nerv. & Ment. Dis. **59**:225, 1924.

Negro, F.: Les syndromes parkinsoniens dans l'intoxication sulfocarbonée, Rev. neurol. **37**:518, 1930.

Neustaedter, M., and Liber, A. F.: Concerning the pathology of parkinsonism (idiopathic, arteriosclerotic and postencephalitic) with a report of 15 necropsies, J. Nerv. & Ment. Dis. **86**:264, 1937.

Nonne, M.: Syphilis und Nervensystem, ed. 5, Berlin, Karger, 1924.

Secrétan, A., and Hedinger, E.: Parkinsonisme après encéphalite léthargique, Schweiz. med. Wchnschr. **8**:937, 1922.

Spatz, H.: Zur Pathogenese und Pathophysiologie der Encephalitis epidemics, Zentralbl. d. ges. Neurol. u. Psychiat. **49**:120, 1924.

Spielmeyer, W.: Zur Pathogenese örtlich elektive Gehirnveränderungen, Zentralbl. d. ges. Neurol. u. Psychiat. **41**:700, 1925.

Stiefler, G.: Striärer Symptomenkomplex als Spätfolge einer im Felde erlittenen Gasvergiftung, Ztschr. d. ges. Neurol. u. Psychiat. **81**:142, 1923.

Trétiakoff, C.: Contribution à l'étude de l'anatomie pathologique du locus niger de Soemmering avec quelques déductions rélatives à la pathogénie des troubles du tonus musculaire de la maladie de parkinson, Thèse de Paris, No. 293, 1919.

Urechia, C. J.: Encéphalite épidémique avec Parkinsonisme et accés transitoires psychomoteurs, Autopsie, Buil. et mém. Soc. méd. hôp. Paris **38**:651, 1922.

————: La syphilis peut-elle reproduire le syndrome de Parkinson, Rev. neurol. **37**:584, 1921.

Vogt, D., and Vogt, O.: Zur Lehre der Erkrankungen des striären Systems, J. Psychol. u. Neurol. **25**:627, 1920.

Wohlwill, F.: Über Gehirnveranderungen bei Leuchtgasvergiftung, Zentralbl. d. ges. Neurol. u. Psychiat. **25**:346, 1921.

5

SYMPTOMATOLOGY

Lewis J. Doshay, M.D.

PARKINSONISM is not a disease in the strict sense, but a symptom complex due to a variety of causes. It was described by Parkinson in his classical treatise of 1817 as follows: "Involuntary tremulous motion, with lessened muscular power, with a propensity to bend the trunk forward and to pass from a walking to a running pace, the senses and intellects being uninjured." It could hardly be better defined today.

The four cardinal symptoms of parkinsonism are rigidity, tremor, akinesia and the loss of spontaneous and automatic movement. These and the sequellae of rigidity, such as the fixed expression, abnormal posture, difficulties of chewing and swallowing, poor balance, impaired gait and weakness and fatigue are common to all types of Parkinson patients. Postencephalitic cases, in addition, may show oculogyria, respiratory tics, lethargy and sialorrhea.

NATURE OF THE SYMPTOMS

Cranial Nerves

Eyes. Pupillary changes in shape, size or reaction to accommodation are present in a high percentage of postencephalitic cases (Table 1). Strabismus is present in about 20 per cent of these cases. Poor ocular convergence is a regular finding in postencephalitic patients and to a much less degree in idiopathic patients. The staring gaze of parkinsonism is in part due to rigidity of the eye muscles and in part to the fixed facies and retraction of the orbicularis oculi.

TABLE 1. SYMPTOMS OF THE THREE TYPES
OF PARKINSONISM*

SYMPTOMS	POSTEN-CEPHALITIC TYPE	IDIO-PATHIC TYPE	ARTERIO-SCLEROTIC TYPE
Lethargy	100%	25%	
Oculogyria	40%		
Strabismus	20%		
Pupillary Abnormalities	75%		
Diplopia	Occasional		
Weakness of Ocular Converg.	100%	25%	
Rigidity	60–70%	70–90%	100%
Tremor	50%	100%	70–90%
Akinesia	100%	50–75%	90–100%
Sialorrhea	100%	25%	10% (?)
Speech Disorders	75–90%	25%	10%
Dysphagia	Occasional	Occasional	25–40%

* As derived from two series of Parkinson cases, each consisting of 100 unselected patients.

Facial Movements. Fixed or masked facies is one of the most frequent symptoms of parkinsonism. The palpebral fissures are wide, and blinking is infrequent. Blepharospasm often appears on attempts to close the eyes. If the forehead is tapped, or if a quick thrust is made toward the eyes, several reflex blinking movements follow (Myerson's sign). Facial movements, whether volitional or emotional, are weak and slow of execution. The lips move sluggishly and in a minimal range, thereby contributing to the poor speech. There may be facial asymmetry on one side.

Speech Disorders. The nasal and monotone quality of speech is in large part due to the difficulty in using the lips and tongue in articulation. Whispering speech occurs among some patients, even when there is no true aphonia or dysphonia. This may be due to lethargy, to indisposition to exert the lung muscles, or to actual rigidity of the respiratory musculature. Not infrequently the speech disorder is of pseudobulbar origin, particularly in arteriosclerotic patients. Repetitive speech is seen occasionally in postencephalitic cases and is probably due to lethargy and lack of attention. Tremulous speech assuming the characteristics of "staccato" is observed at times in patients where tremor has acquired major proportions. In a small percentage of patients speech is so badly impaired, that it is almost impossible to understand them.

Chewing and Swallowing. In cases with advanced rigidity of the masseter muscles, chewing may be slow and labored. At times swallowing, especially of solid foods, may also be impaired, whether because of rigidity, pseudobulbar weakness, or a combination of both. In many, reflex swallowing is lost or sluggish and contributes to the tendency to drool, especially during sleep, or in the erect posture with the head drooping. Other cranial nerve functions (taste, smell, vision, etc.) are unaffected by the Parkinson illness, but may be by drugs or intercurrent situations.

Posture, Balance and Gait

Posture. Many abnormal postures occur among

Parkinson patients, not the least uncommon of which are the bent posture of the head, the stooped posture of the trunk, the forward roll of the shoulders, the adduction of the arms, flexion and pronation of the forearms and the pill-rolling position of the fingers. The distortion of body posture is in general related to the stronger force of the flexors of the neck, trunk, arm and calf, to the stronger pull of the adductors of the thigh and the greater strength of the pronators of the forearm. Rigidity, the supervening contractures and the greater involvement of one side of the body are contributing factors. Faulty postures severely impair motion, balance and gait.

Balance. Advanced rigidity, akinesia and faulty postures render proper balance difficult for some patients, when walking or standing. There is lack of agility and speed in adjusting the muscles necessary to upright equilibratory co-ordination. The adduction of the thighs leads to walking on a narrow base, which adds to poor body balance.

Gait. Rigidity of the calf muscles with shortening of the tendo achillis leads to a talipes equino varus foot, so that the patient walks on his toes. The body is thrown forward, past the center of gravity, and a *festinating and propulsive gait* develops. The patient is forced to make rapid steps in an effort to catch up with his line of gravity. He occasionally succeeds by a sudden straightening of the trunk, but most often the force of gravity and the weight of body pull him forward, until he stops himself against a wall, some object, or falls to the floor. Soon or late, such patients become dependent upon others for safety in standing or walking. Occasionally, a retropulsive gait develops from rigidity of the extensor spinal muscles. Some elderly rigid patients employ a shuffling gait, the so-called *marche-à-petits-pas.* The body moves en masse, with short steps and absent swing in the arms.

Motor System

Weakness and Fatigue. Frequently one of the earliest complaints is tiredness and weakness. Rigidity, like the brakes on a wheel, opposes motion, so that greater effort is necessary for the patient to perform his daily chores. This leads to an increased feeling of fatigue and weakness. Weakness is also pronounced on arising, probably because of lack of muscular movement during sleep and the increased rigidity occasioned thereby. It is interesting, nevertheless, that some patients with fairly pronounced rigidity find it possible to perform a full day's work without unusual fatigue. Disuse may bring some general wasting of the musculature, but focal atrophies rarely occur. Fibrillations are not a feature of the illness.

Akinesia (Poverty and Slowness of Movement). The cause of sluggishness of movement or akinesia is not clearly understood, and it cannot be attributed entirely to rigidity, because many patients, especially the postencephalitic and idiopathic types, show little rigidity and yet move very slowly. The poorness of automatic movement may contribute but does not fully account for the akinesia. In some patients, perhaps lethargy and other mental components may be partly responsible.

Loss of Associated, Automatic and Spontaneous Movement. This is one of the earliest signs of the illness. It is present in varying degree in different patients, and one of its mildest forms is manifested in the reduced swing of one arm during walking. However, careful scrutiny will disclose that the deficit operates in almost every action of the patient. He does not rise spontaneously or lift his cup automatically, or talk, walk or write freely. Every move is preceded by a pause, until voluntary activation takes effect. In more advanced cases, the patient sits like a statue—the eyelids never blink; the lips hardly budge; the neck and shoulders never shift for a second; the trunk does not move to right or left; and the legs remain motionless. This may go on for minutes or more until, because of discomfort in the muscles, he makes a limited voluntary change in position, or requests someone to shift him. At times, the latter proves exasperating for the family, since some advanced patients repeat the demand every few seconds.

Rigidity. The rigidity of parkinsonism differs from the hypertonicity of pyramidal lesions in that it is present to an equal degree in opposing muscle groups, for example, the flexors and the extensors of the knee. In pyramidal conditions, the hypertonicity is more prominent in the flexors of the arm and the extensors of the leg. Moreover, rigidity differs from spasticity in that it persists throughout the entire range of movement at any joint and yields to pressure or pull in an interrupted series of successive steps or jerks, from which the term "cogwheel" rigidity is derived. By contrast, a spastic limb yields to greater force than its own resistance by a sudden collapse in "clasp-knife" fashion. Rigidity may be of mild degree and limited to one side so that it hardly interferes with work, and only slight progression appears in the course of many years, while in other cases rigidity tends to spread rapidly from the afflicted side to the other side of the body and may progress to severe proportions. In a very few Parkinson cases with no tremor, a "plastic" or leathery type of rigidity is found.

A most disturbing complication of rigidity is *contracture*. Rigidity tends to limit the use of the affected parts. Disuse leads to myofibrosis and shortening of the muscles, which in turn render movement still more difficult. Thus a vicious cycle develops that can lead to a progression of contractures and deformities, so that ultimately the patient can scarcely move and has to be confined to a chair or his bed.

Contractures may develop in any muscles of the body, but the most common sites are the neck, shoulders, elbows, fingers, hips, knees and ankles. The neck flexors shorten and pull the head forward and downward. The flexors of the spine similarly pull the body forward. Contractures in the arm adductors lead to freezing of the shoulder joint, with or without benefit of original or secondary osteoarthritis. Contractures in the pronators and the flexors of the arm often bring the upper limbs into a flexed position across the groin and interfere with walking. The fingers may show contractures in the flexor and adductor muscles which serve to limit the small movements employed in writing, buttoning of clothes, cutting food, etc.

Tremor. Tremor in parkinsonism is produced by rhythmical, alternating movements of the opposing muscle groups of a joint. Generally the hand is the segment first and most affected. The tremor here may be in the nature of a flexion and extension of the wrist, or supination and pronation, or a lateral displacement. When the fingers are involved, the movement is mostly at the metacarpophalangeal joints, giving, when the thumb participates, the effect of a "pill-rolling" motion. Less frequently, the tremor is confined to the elbow and the shoulder.

In the lower extremities the tremor is generally less

marked and in the majority of cases can be noted only in a sitting or reclining position. One or both ankles may show a flexion and extension movement of the foot, which is sometimes transmitted to the knee. Tremor of the head is not commonly seen and consists of flexion and extension, or a lateral oscillation. Occasionally, tremor of the jaw may appear as a rhythmic vertical or lateral displacement and may be accompanied by tremor of the tongue, or the latter may exist independently. Tremor may be confined to one or a few joints or be almost generalized. The bilateral, continuous and severe form of tremor is often associated with sweating, loss of weight and appetite and insomnia.

The tremor of parkinsonism is of the resting type. It has a frequency of 4 to 6 beats per second. In most cases it disappears or diminishes for a short time, when the patient performs a voluntary act. Frequently, patients can also diminish or stop tremor at will for short periods of time. Tremor disappears with sleep, or in the twilight state before and after. It also disappears under general anesthesia.

Tremor may be the first symptom to appear in parkinsonism but in many cases it is preceded by akinesia, weakness, or rigidity, especially among the older arteriosclerotic patients. The postencephalitic tremor is a trace slower than that of the idiopathic or arteriosclerotic types. In some cases the postencephalitic tremor gives the impression of being somewhat more complex, having some athetoid features.

Tremor is greatly influenced by emotional factors, increasing when the patient is tense, fearful or anxious, and diminishing when he is in good spirits. At times without any obvious reason, but probably due to hidden psychological factors, tremor as well as the other symptoms of parkinsonism may improve for days, weeks or even months and then, under apparently optimum conditions, return to its previous status. A few patients have little or no visible tremor but complain of internal, visceral or abdominal tremor.

Sensory System

All modalities of sensation are preserved in parkinsonism. Pains in muscles and joints and cramps are frequently complained of by patients and are probably due to rigidity, contracture and joint changes.

Reflexes

Usually there are no changes in reflexes in parkinsonism, but they may be difficult to elicit in some patients on account of the rigidity, or they may appear different on the two sides because of varying degrees of rigidity.

Only when there is damage to the pyramidal system, as often happens in arteriosclerotic cases, may a change of reflexes take place, along with a Babinski sign.

Autonomic Nervous System

Sialorrhea is a common symptom of postencephalitic parkinsonism and to a lesser degree occurs among idiopathic cases. Drooling occurs not so much because of excess saliva as because of weakness of pharyngeal muscles, the loss of reflex swallowing of the saliva and the flexed position of the head, which allows the saliva to pour out across the chin. Occasionally patients complain of episodes of profuse perspiration on arising or at other times of the day. Parkinson patients are sensitive to changes in weather and frequently feel very uncomfortable during the warm season. An oily skin is often seen among post-encephalitic patients, as well as a slow pulse and low blood pressure, as part of the general sluggish metabolism.

Mental Symptoms

Odd forms of behavior were common features of postencephalitic cases, especially juveniles, during the 1920 decade, but are rarely seen these days. Depression is a common finding among the advanced cases. As in other chronic diseases, it is a reaction to the disabilities caused by the illness. Some despondent patients attempt suicide and, if they do not succeed, terminate in State Hospitals. An occasional patient may show a paranoid trend. Terminal cases may manifest confusion, delirium and lethargy, before passing into coma.

Often patients with advanced rigidity of the limbs complain of spells of being "glued" or "frozen" to the ground. This is frequently induced by the challenge of having to do something hurriedly and the fear of incapacity to do so. The process seems to be a sudden, generalized, muscular spasm. The patient stands transfixed and helpless for a minute or more, when the limbs suddenly loosen and he is able to move again.

TYPES OF PARKINSONISM

Patients with parkinsonism can be divided into three main groups: postencephalitic, idiopathic and arteriosclerotic. This classification is probably not the ideal, but considering what is known about parkinsonism, it is the most rational from the clinical and therapeutic points of view. The different types can be easily differentiated (Table 2). Treatment varies somewhat with each type (Bremer, 1925; Doshay, 1953). Parkinsonism may also develop secondarily to injury of the basal ganglia, by carbon monoxide poisoning, manganese poisoning, syphilis, tumors of the brain and in association with Wilson's and other heredodegenerative diseases, but these are of comparatively rare occurrence.

Postencephalitic Parkinsonism

Under this group are included cases due to encephalitis of the Von Economo type, that developed their symptoms shortly or many years after the acute episode. The vast majority of postencephalitic cases seen today are casualties of the epidemics of 1918-1928, although a few sporadic cases have appeared since. Some of the cases have no history of encephalitis, but are classified on clinical grounds.

The Parkinsonian symptoms may appear at any time after the episode of influenza or encephalitis, but generally set in 5, 10, or even 20 years after the acute illness. The age of onset is usually between 20 and 30 and rarely if ever after 40 years. The patient is hardly conscious of exactly when his illness began, but on careful questioning, he or his relatives may recall that for several months or years there had been a slowing down of movement and speech, with a slight dragging of one foot, or a mild tremor of the hands when nervous. Further questioning may reveal an easy tendency to sleep, noticeable for many years in the past. Often there is a clearcut history of influenza or encephalitis in childhood, characterized by several days to several weeks of coma, delirium, or mental confusion and

TABLE 2. DIFFERENCES AMONG THE THREE TYPES OF PARKINSONISM

CHARACTERISTICS	POSTENCEPHALITIC TYPE	IDIOPATHIC TYPE	ARTERIOSCLEROTIC TYPE
Age of Onset	20-35	40-55	55-70
Sex	Male—61% Female—39%	Male—67% Female—33%	Male—62% Female—38%
Past History	Influenza Encephalitis	Good Health	Hypertension Cerebral Vascular Episodes Giddiness, Tinnitus Cardiovascular Disease
Prodromata	Lethargy Sluggishness Sialorrhea Montone Speech	None	Akinesia Tiredness
Type of Onset	Evanescent	Sudden	Evanescent
First Symptoms	Rigidity and Postural Abnormality or Oculogyria	Tremor	Rigidity
Distribution of Symptoms	Diffuse	Hemi-involvement	Hemi-involvement
Nature of Symptoms	Lethargy, Diplopia Oculogyria, Strabismus Pupil Abnormalities Weak Eye Convergence Rigidity, Akinesia Tremor, Sialorrhea Loss of Spontaneity	Tremor Rigidity Sialorrhea Somnolence Montone Speech	Rigidity, Akinesia Tremor Dysphagia
Course of Symptoms	Progressive, but very slowly, with long stationary phases	Slowly progressive	Progression is often rapid

followed by transient diplopia, strabismus, oculogyria, sialorrhea and sleep abnormalities (von Witzleben, 1942). Caution should be used against the hasty conclusion that every Parkinson under 40 who gives a history of "influenza" is a postencephalitic case.

The acute phase is followed by a short or long interval of relative "normalcy," during which time the only manifestation of the underlying condition appears in the form of periodic drowsiness and a ready tendency to fall asleep. Then the early symptoms of parkinsonism, akinesia, tiredness and increasing somnolence become noticeable. This is followed in a year or more by rigidity of the limbs on the same or opposite sides. The fixed facies, monotone speech, posturing of the neck and trunk and sialorrhea also become apparent. Tremor is a later development.

The rigidity is usually of mild degree and may remain stationary for 10 or 20 years, with help of therapy, and then progress to severe and disabling proportions, or there may be little progression in rigidity, but tremor may be added.

In about 40 per cent of postencephalitic cases, the initial symptom is in the nature of oculogyric crises, which may be the only complaint presented by the patient. These may occur from several times a day to once in many weeks. The eyes generally turn upward and remain there for minutes to 12 hours or more. At times, regardless of what is done for the patient, the spell will not end until he falls asleep. In some cases the crises disappear spontaneously, or with the help of drugs, after several years.

Strabismus appears in some 20 per cent of cases and is usually of mild degree. A history of diplopia following the acute phase is often elicited. This may last from one to several years, with subsequent milder and transient episodes. Varying degrees of weakness of ocular convergence are found in almost all cases. A high percentage show irregular or unequal pupils. The light reflex is usually well preserved, but accommodation is impaired, due to the weakness of convergence.

Torticollis, dystonic movements of tongue, face and arms and myoclonic movements of the pharynx are relatively infrequent complications. However, lethargy of varying degree is common to almost every patient. Narcolepsy is present in a small percentage of cases.

Idiopathic Parkinsonism

This type sets in at 40 to 55 years of age, and generally the onset is characterized by the sudden appearance of tremor of one extremity in a background of previous good health. Frequently, careful examination will establish a slight amount of rigidity in the arm and the leg and some asymmetry of the face on the same side (hemiparkinsonism).

The condition progresses, and in a year or two there are clear-cut signs of cogwheel rigidity and an increase in tremor. Soon after, the condition passes to the other side of the face, and the expression becomes fixed. Within perhaps another year, the rigidity spreads to the neck and trunk and then to the limbs of the other side of the body. Sialorrhea, monotone speech, slight weakness of ocular convergence and some somnolence appear in a small percentage of cases.

In women, idiopathic parkinsonism frequently begins at the menopause. In some patients the onset of illness is preceded by an acute emotional or traumatic episode, such as a death in the family, the loss of a job, an operation, etc., and they tend to attribute to these happenings a causal relationship.

Arteriosclerotic Parkinsonism

This variety rarely sets in before 55 years of age and most commonly after 60. Unlike the abrupt and dramatic onset of the idiopathic type, the onset here is usually evanescent, with a creeping type of rigidity and akinesia affecting all the limbs, but more marked on one side of the body than on the other. The face shows early masking, while the neck and the trunk assume a fixed posture, with some flexion and stooping. The gait soon becomes the *marche-à-petits-pas*. Tremor does not appear until a year or two later and it may grow to severe proportions. The rigidity may progress to contractures in the limbs and lead to a festinating gait, to inability to walk without assistance and to the need of a wheelchair. Finally, the patient may become bedridden and be subject to pressure sores and other complications.

Usually, throughout the course, the eyes remain "sharp" and the mind alert, but in a few cases psychosis due to arteriosclerosis with periods of disorientation and confusion may occur. In most cases there is no sign of somnolence or lethargy, unless vast areas of the brain become softened by the arteriosclerotic process, during the terminal stages of illness.

Younger hypertensive arteriosclerotic cases may show an abrupt onset of Parkinson symptoms, possibly related to one or more cerebral vascular insults, but the older arteriosclerotic cases with low blood pressure commonly have a gradual onset. Pesudobulbar signs may appear in the form of difficulties of speech, chewing and swallowing. Unilateral pyramidal signs are often found with hyperreflexia and Babinski sign. Sensory modalities are rarely impaired.

DIAGNOSTIC SIGNS AND TESTS

Diagnostic Signs

The diagnosis of advanced parkinsonism is obvious. In early cases a more careful examination is required, but in general the diagnosis is relatively easy, if one pays attention to the following signs:

1. *Spiked Knuckles.* If a trace of rigidity is present in a patient, it will make its earliest appearance at the metacarpophalangeal joints as a slight hump when the hands are extended. The sign is particularly helpful because in the early stages of illness only one side is affected, so that the spiked knuckles of the abnormal hand stand out prominently, in comparison with the normal side.

2. *Adiadokokinesis.* This is likewise one of the surest and very earliest signs of parkinsonism. In testing the hands for succession movements in the outstretched position, the affected limb always lags behind the normal. The movement is sluggish, awkward and tends to tire very quickly, as compared with the normal.

3. *Cogwheel.* This jerky resistance to passive movement of a joint appears very early in the illness, especially at the wrist. Several trials of movement will bring out some traces of cogwheel in an affected limb, and comparisons should be made with the normal side.

4. *Absent Swing of the Arm.* The absence of associated swing in an affected arm during walking is easy to observe, even in cases where rigidity is not detectable. The affected limb does not swing in rhythm with

the opposite leg. Comparison can be made with the swing of the normal arm. The sign is brought out more sharply if the patient is asked to walk on heels or toes.

5. *Fixity of Expression.* This is a fairly early sign that can almost always be found among postencephalitic cases and to a lesser extent among idiopathic and arteriosclerotic cases. The retraction of the orbicularis oculi, the infrequent blinking, the staring gaze, the lack of play in the facial muscles and the lack of movement in the forehead and eyebrows render this sign easy of recognition.

6. *Monotone Speech.* This type of indistinct speech has a nasal quality and is easy to recognize. It appears fairly early in the illness.

7. *Sialorrhea.* Excessive salivation, and especially drooling on the pillow at night, is a common and very early symptom of parkinsonism. Its absence at the time of the examination may be due to the use of one of the belladonna preparations, and this should be inquired into.

8. *Weakness of Ocular Convergence.* This is commonly found in postencephalitic cases and in some idiopathic cases, but rarely if ever in the arteriosclerotic type.

9. *Rhythmic Alternating Tremor.* When present, the characteristic tremor at rest with a frequency of from 4 to 6 per second, which diminishes or stops on voluntary or purposeful movements, makes parkinsonism easily distinguishable from other diseases. In idiopathic cases this may be the earliest and often the only presenting sign.

10. *Wartenberg's Sign.* The patient is placed at the edge of a table with the legs hanging freely. The ex-

aminer lifts the legs simultaneously to the same horizontal plane, then suddenly releases them. In a normal
person, the legs swing 6 or 7 times after displacement,
whereas in parkinsonism the number of swings is reduced. The sign is especially helpful if only one side
is affected, so that ready comparisons can be made
with the normal limb (Wartenberg, 1951).

Diagnostic Tests

The results of routine laboratory tests in parkinsonism are generally within normal limits. The basal
metabolic rate is lowered in the lethargic patient and
higher in cases with severe tremor as a major feature.
The serum cholesterol is often elevated. The spinal
fluid protein is slightly increased in some cases. The
electro-encephalogram does not show any consistent
abnormality. The electrocardiogram may be abnormal
in arteriosclerotic cases, with coronary disease.

The electromyogram is of diagnostic value in early
and doubtful cases. The records of parkinsonism differ
from those of normally innervated muscles, as well as
from those of other diseases of the nervous system.

In patients with rigidity and no visible tremor, the
electromyograph records taken with surface or coaxial
needle electrodes show in muscles at rest a continuous
influx of low-voltage action potentials (Fig. 15 A). On
active movement (Fig. 15 B) and passive movement
(Fig. 15 C), there is a grouping of the action potentials in rhythmic bursts, at the rate of about 4 to 6
per second, which replace the continuous influx of
the resting muscle. Fig. 15 D shows that these bursts
of activity correspond with the "cogwheel" phenomenon. The EMG also shows that in parkinsonism, when
two leads are derived from the same muscle at rest,

as well as on passive or active movement, there is a marked tendency to synchronization of the electrical activity, in contrast with that found in normal muscle.

In patients with tremor, the EMG records (Fig. 15 E) reveal that the number of spikes in an individual burst, their amplitude and their duration vary greatly in different parts of the same record, but the frequency of the bursts is more or less constant for all muscles of the same patient. However, slight variation occurs from patient to patient. Fig. 15 F shows that the rhythmic bursts of synchronous activity occur at the rate of about 4 to 6 per second, separated by intervals of no electrical activity, or low voltage continuous activity. The bursts of action potentials in the protagonists regularly alternate with those of the antagonists, and thereby the rhythmic tremor of parkinsonism takes place.

DIFFERENTIAL DIAGNOSIS

Usually the diagnosis of parkinsonism is not difficult, but an occasional case may be mistaken for multiple sclerosis, brain tumor, etc. The diagnostic signs of parkinsonism will serve to differentiate early doubtful cases, and the electromyogram can be of added help.

Multiple Sclerosis. Intention tremor and nystagmus are common, as well as pyramidal and posterior column signs. The cogwheel phenomenon is absent.

Brain Tumor. There may be hebetude and sluggishness in a patient with brain tumor, but no rhythmic tremor, cogwheel rigidity, or masked facies.

Wilson's Disease. This is familial and usually sets in at an early age. Tremor is often absent at rest, but

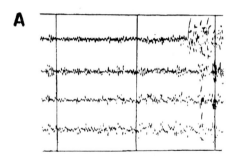

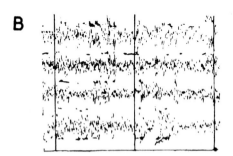

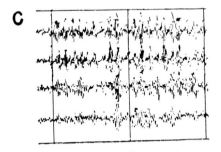

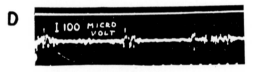

E

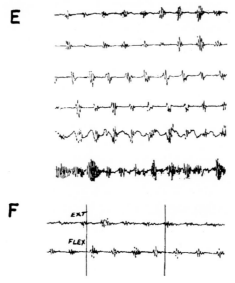

F

FIG. 15. (A) Rigid muscle antagonists at rest. Two pairs of electrodes from the biceps (upper half of the record) and two from the triceps (lower half of the record). At end of record, active movement begins. (B) Continuation of record (active movement of biceps and triceps). (C) Passive extension, otherwise as in A and B. (D) "Staccato" (cogwheel) movement brought out by active or passive movement; very similar to tremor bursts. A to C were taken with inkwriting oscillograph; time, 1 second between vertical lines. D, with cathode ray oscillograph; time, 1/60 of a second between white dots at bottom of record. (E) Record taken from a variety of muscles of both arms and right leg. (F) Antagonist muscles in alternating tremor. E and F inkwriting oscillograph. Time in F is 1 second between lines. (Paul F. A. Hoefer)

71

when the arms are outstretched it can become violent (wing-beating). The rhythm is more rapid (5 to 7 beats a second). Other signs, such as the Kaiser-Fleischer ring and hepatitis, serve to establish the diagnosis.

Familial Tremor. This starts in early childhood. There is usually a family history. Rigidity and other signs of parkinsonism are absent. The tremor is generally of fine type but may become irregular in amplitude under effort and emotion.

Senile Tremor. This generally consists of a lateral head oscillation. In cases where the tremor involves the arms, the amplitude is much finer than in parkinsonism and often disappears at rest. There is no rigidity, akinesia, or postural abnormality. The onset is generally later than in arteriosclerotic parkinsonism.

Carbon Monoxide Encephalopathy. This shows evidence of *severe* cortical involvement, in addition to the basal ganglia signs. The patients are usually disoriented for time and place and show poor ability to concentrate or calculate. As a rule, Parkinson patients are mentally well preserved.

General Paresis. The tremor is characteristically perioral and when present in the hands and the arms is of fine type. The mental changes, serology and Argyll Robertson pupils serve to differentiate it.

Manganese Encephalopathy. There is usually a history of industrial exposure. Hepatic cirrhosis is frequently present. Pseudobulbar features are prominent. Tremor is chiefly of the head and much finer than in parkinsonism. Memory and other mental faculties are impaired, although recovery of the same is greater than in carbon monoxide poisoning.

COURSE AND PROGNOSIS

In the majority of cases the symptoms progress slowly for many years. A few show a rapid, downhill course of 2 or 3 years. Many of them become disabled soon or late, but even in this condition with good care they can live for another 5 or 10 years. Death is usually due to intercurrent illnesses.

Treatment with drugs, psychotherapy and physiotherapy, and living an active life have an effect in retarding the progression of the symptoms. About 90 per cent of Parkinson patients are ambulatory and can obtain reasonably good treatment at a clinic or a private office. The other 10 per cent are advanced and disabled cases that cannot travel or reach treatment facilities with any regularity and deteriorate from neglect.

Postencephalitic Type. Oculogyric crises may be the only presenting symptom for 10 to 20 years, and then usually rigidity is added, progressing slowly over a period of years, or proceeding rapidly to contractures, postural deformities, weakness, invalidism, cachexia and an exitus through some minor complicating illness. In other cases, the oculogyric crises disappear after several years. Stationary periods, lasting 10 or more years during which no manifest change in the symptoms takes place, are not rare. Some patients are unable to perform gainful work, more because of their mental status (obsessive-compulsive features, lethargy and emotional lability) than the progression of the disease.

Idiopathic Type. Here also the course may be slowly

or rapidly progressive, but it is usually longer than that of the arteriosclerotic type. More years of useful working ability can be expected than in encephalitic cases. The age of onset seems to have some influence on the course of the disease, and patients whose first symptoms set in early in life progress slower than those with a late onset. Stationary periods lasting from 3 to 10 years or more are not unusual in this type of parkinsonism. Tremor and rigidity may remain a long time on one side of the body before they pass to the other, and even then the picture may or may not progress rapidly. Many cases in the seventh decade, or before, commence to show signs of cerebral arteriosclerosis, and from then on their course is not unlike that of the arteriosclerotic type.

Arteriosclerotic Type. Usually rigidity and akinesia are bilateral almost from the start. Tremor appears a number of years later and then it often becomes of major proportions. Stationary phases of 3 to 5 years in duration may occur. The symptoms usually progress much more rapidly than in the other two groups and lead to contractures, deformities and pains and aches in muscles and joints, which at times are highly aggravating to the patient and his family.

If the arteriosclerotic changes affect the cortex, episodes of disorientation, confusion, or psychosis may supervene (psychosis with cerebral arteriosclerosis). At 75 or 80, they may show progression in the cerebral arteriosclerosis, with thromboses and diffuse cerebral infarction, and pass into coma, sometimes preceded by a stroke. Or, as in other chronic disabling neurologic diseases, death may come at an earlier age from complications, such as pneumonia.

REFERENCES

Bremer, F. W.: High atropine tolerance in postencephalitic parkinsonism, Deutsches Arch. f. Klin. Med. **149**:340, 1925.

Doshay, L. J.: Parkinsonism (postencephalitic, idiopathic and arteriosclerotic), Current Therapy, Saunders, Philadelphia, 1953, p. 652.

Parkinson, J.: An essay on the shaking palsy, Sherwood, Neely and Jones, 1817.

Wartenberg, R.: Pendulousness of the legs as a diagnostic test, Neurology **1**:18, 1951.

Witzleben, von, H. D.: Methods of Treatment in Postencephalitic Parkinsonism, p. 22, New York, Grune, 1942.

6

DRUG THERAPY

Lewis J. Doshay, M.D.
Adolfo Zier, M.D.

THE exact number of patients with parkinsonism is unknown, but the disease must be very common, since it is estimated by Goodman (Fig. 16) as third in the list of major disabling conditions. The burden of care of the vast majority of these people falls upon the general practitioner, who sees them from the onset of illness. This is the time when the greatest good can be accomplished, through a proper orientation of the patient toward his illness and the setting of a suitable program of therapy.

Early and intensive treatment can insure these patients many years of productive life. It should then be obvious why the family physician has to keep abreast of the recent advances in therapy. Moreover, in doing so, he may be pleasantly surprised to find that parkinsonism is actually one of the easiest and most gratifying illnesses to treat, because the patients expect very little and are appreciative of any betterment in their condition.

To provide an up-to-the-minute picture of the chemotherapy of parkinsonism will be the aim of this chapter. It should be understood, however, that medicinal therapy is but part of the treatment, and in most cases

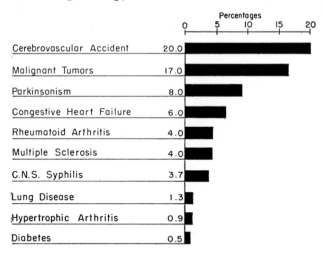

Percentages

Cerebrovascular Accident	20.0
Malignant Tumors	17.0
Parkinsonism	8.0
Congestive Heart Failure	6.0
Rheumatoid Arthritis	4.0
Multiple Sclerosis	4.0
C.N.S. Syphilis	3.7
Lung Disease	1.3
Hypertrophic Arthritis	0.9
Diabetes	0.5

Fig. 16. Major disabling conditions among chronic diseases. (Based upon an analysis of 431 patients admitted to the Cleveland Nursing Home between January, 1946, and July, 1952—J. I. Goodman, J. A. M. A., **152**:1336, 1953.)

it has to be combined with psychotherapy and physical therapy.

DRUGS IN CURRENT USE

The medicinal treatment of parkinsonism has made vast strides during the past ten years (Doshay and Constable, 1951). Prior to that, the solanaceous plant extracts and their congeners, hyoscine, stramonium, atropine, Rabellon, Bellabulgara and Vinobel, were the only preparations of value. Since then, and especially within the last five years, a host of synthetic drugs have become available. In fact, their number is growing so rapidly, that it has become difficult for the busy general practitioner to keep up with them. The drugs in common use will therefore be presented individually, with comments on their structure, actions, side effects and method of administration.

Potato Plant Products

Hyoscine (scopolamine). This is an extract of the solanaceous or potato family plants, especially stramonium and scopola. For its structural formula, see Figure 17. It is available in 1/200 gr. (0.3 mg.), 1/150 gr. (0.45 mg.) and 1/100 gr. (0.6 mg.) white tablets (Plate 1). Older patients fare better on 1/200 gr. doses and younger patients on the 1/150 or 1/100 gr. doses, two or three times a day. Hyoscine is exactly the same as scopolamine, which name is associated with an old method of extraction. Hyoscine is the best current drug for the control of tremor, tension, agitation and excitement in Parkinson patients (Epidemic Encephalitis, 1939). The side reactions most commonly complained of by patients are somnolence, "dopiness," dryness of the mouth and blurred vision. It is a common observation that the side effects of drowsiness, which pass entirely unnoticed in encephalitic cases, can prove highly disturbing to arteriosclerotic patients because of their general hypersensitiveness to drugs. Dexedrine in 2½ mg. doses sometimes helps to counteract this untoward reaction.

Atropine Solution (0.5 per cent). Atropine is the chief alkaloid of belladonna, and its structural formula appears in Figure 17. The solution is a colorless liquid. It is inexpensive, and since it tends to deteriorate on standing, a fresh supply should be obtained each month. The prescription is simple to write—atropine sulfate gr. V to aqua dest. oz. ii. The druggist should

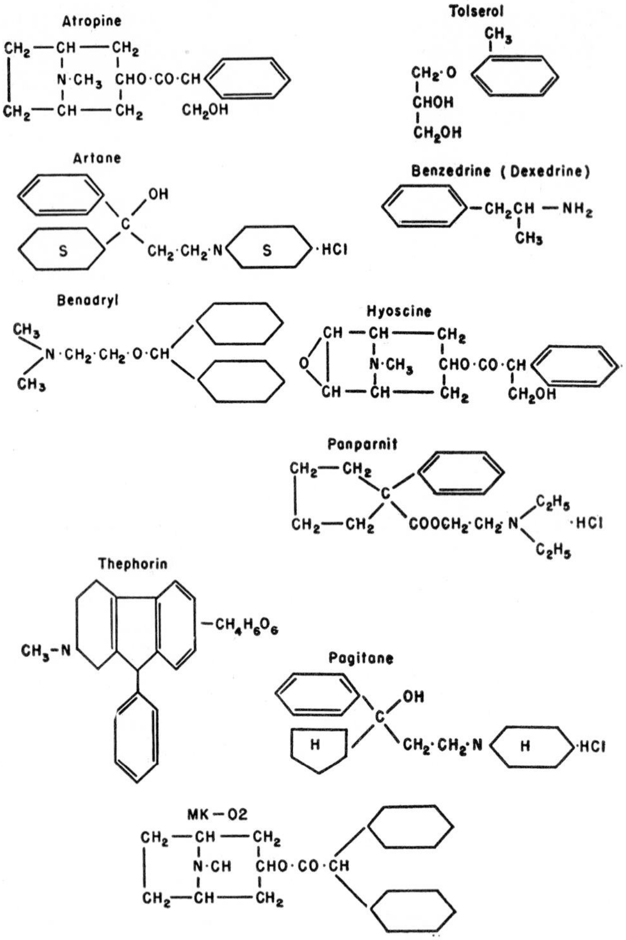

FIG. 17. The structural formula of drugs employed in parkinsonism.

be asked to provide a special dropper measuring one minim to each drop. It is administered in 3 drop

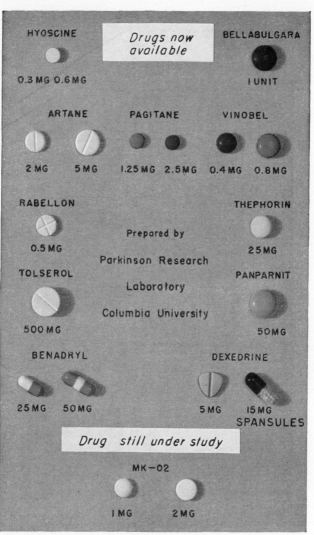

PLATE 1

The most common drugs employed in the treatment of parkinsonism.

doses t.i.d., with an interval of six hours between medication. The dose should be increased one drop t.i.d.
every three days, until the optimum dose is reached.
It is rarely necessary to go beyond ten drops, except for
the control of oculogyria, when the dose may be elevated to 15 drops t.i.d. The 0.5 per cent solution
makes easy calculation, since three drops are equal to
1 mg. of atropine or roughly 1/60 of a grain; 10 drops
to 3 mg. or 1/20 of a grain; 15 drops to 5 mg. or 1/12
of a grain, etc. Atropine is an excellent remedy for the
postencephalitic and some of the younger idiopathic
cases (Neal, 1934; Adams and Hays, 1933; Roemer,
1931; Kleeman, 1929). It is a powerful relaxant for
spasm, rigidity and contracture, but has practically no
action against tremor, for which hyoscine has to be
added. Because of the hazard of glaucoma and other
disturbing side reactions, *it should never be dispensed
to arteriosclerotic patients.* Side reactions within therapeutic dosage are dryness of the mouth, blurring of
vision, and occasionally nausea, palpitation and flush-
ing of the face and chest. In excess dosage, it can produce nausea, vomiting, dizziness, mental confusion and
hallucinations. Atropine is the essential agent of Bellabulgara, Vinobel, Rabellon and belladonna (Doshay,
1942).

Stramonium. This natural product is obtained
from the leaves of the potato plant, *Datura stramonium,* and is generally employed in the form of the
tincture. It contains atropine, hyoscyamine and hyoscine, and exerts a strong action against tremor (von
Witzleben, 1942). The drug is well tolerated by elderly patients. It should be started in 15 drop doses
t.i.d. and slowly increased to 60 drops t.i.d. Thereafter the maintenance dose should fluctuate between

30 and 60 drops. Dryness of the mouth is less than with hyoscine or atropine, and the somnorific reaction is minimal. Davies, Rose & Co. has on the market a grayish-green, egg-shaped, $2\frac{1}{2}$ gr. tablet of the leaves of stramonium, which some patients prefer because it saves the trouble of counting drops. Two to six of these tablets can be used per day.

Bellabulgara. This is an extract of the root of Bulgarian belladonna. It was originally believed that the Bulgarian variety was superior to other belladonna products, but this has long since been disproved. Bellabulgara is manufactured by Lederle Laboratories in one unit, chocolate covered tablets (Plate 1), containing 0.45 mg. of the alkaloids, atropine and hyoscyamine, as well as a trace of hyoscine. Hyoscyamine becomes transformed into atropine immediately after entering the stomach (Sollman, 1936). Bellabulgara is administered in half or full tablet doses t.i.d. It is a good muscle relaxant and has a slight action against tremor. However, since hyoscyamine becomes transformed into atropine, the total content of the pill is less than 1/2 mg. of atropine, which is far below the minimum dose required to maintain postencephalitic cases. It is therefore seldom used alone, except in cases where a mild preparation is needed. The side reactions are dryness of the mouth and blurring of vision (Alcock and Carmichael, 1938; Hill, 1938).

Vinobel. This is a root extract of domestic belladonna and is manufactured by William S. Merrell Company. It is available in two forms; a dark red tablet containing 0.4 mg. of the active alkaloids and a pink tablet containing 0.8 mg. of the same (Plate 1). The two sizes are of advantage in therapy, the larger tablet being more suited to younger patients and the smaller one to older patients. Two to six tablets may be used per day. It has the same actions and side effects as Bellabulgara (Price and Merritt, 1941).

Rabellon. This contains the alkaloids of domestic belladonna in about the same proportion as Bellabulgara and Vinobel. It is manufactured by Sharp & Dohme Laboratories, in the form of a white, double-scored tablet (Plate 1). This is of advantage in therapy, since it can be administered in quarter, half, or full tablets. The full tablet contains 0.5 mg. of the alkaloids. Some patients take as many as eight or ten tablets a day. Even so, ten tablets are equal to but 15 minims of the 1/2 per cent atropine solution or 5 mg. for the day, which is still below the maintenance dose of atropine in postencephalitic cases. It is therefore best used as a supplement to other drugs, or in smaller dosage among older patients. Bellabulgara, Vinobel and Rabellon are well tolerated by elderly patients, in doses of two or three tablets per day, and no case of glaucoma has ever come to our attention from their use in arteriosclerotic patients (Vollmer, 1939; Neal and Dillenberg, 1940).

Belladonna. The preparation is generally employed in the form of the tincture, which is derived from the leaves of belladonna plants. It is administered in 15 drop doses t.i.d., which are slowly increased to 30 drops t.i.d. It is of some value in overcoming rigidity, but has minimal action against tremor (Shapiro, 1952). It must not be dispensed to arteriosclerotic patients, since for reasons unclear, there is a hazard of glaucoma; two such instances have come to our attention. Its use in parkinsonism has largely been displaced by safer and better preparations.

Synthetic Antispasmodics

Artane *(trihexyphenidyl).* This synthetic has the structural formula of 3-(1-piperidyl)-1-phenyl-1-cyclo-hexyl-1-propanol hydrochloride (Fig. 17). It is manufactured by Lederle Laboratories and is available in scored white tablets of 2 and 5 mg. (Plate 1). It is administered in 1 or 2 mg. doses three or four times a day to older patients, and in 5 mg. doses t.i.d. to younger ones. For oculogyric crises, 10 mg. t.i.d. is used. The drug is gentle in action and is well tolerated at all age levels (Doshay, 1949). Its usual side effects are slight dryness (12 per cent of atropine) and blurring of vision. It is our current best preparation for the sustained control of rigidity and its complications (Corbin, 1949; Dow and Rosenbaum, 1949; Ellenbogen, 1950; Phillips, 1950) and should be employed as the basic drug in commencing treatment with new cases. It also has a favorable action against minor tremor (Doshay, 1953). It is a remarkably effective cerebral stimulant and physical activator against sluggishness, fatigue, weakness and akinesia. The action lasts four to six hours. Artane has no pressor action like Benzedrine, and is therefore safe to use in old people. In oculogyria, it is almost a specific and controls or abolishes the spells in 84 per cent of cases (Doshay, to be published). Not more than 10 mg. a day should be given to arteriosclerotic patients; this should preferably be dispensed in $2\frac{1}{2}$ mg. doses four times a day, rather than 5 mg. b.i.d., in order to obviate cerebral excitation, confusion, delirium and hallucinations. These disappear in a day or two upon discontinuation of the drug.

Panparnit *(caramiphen).* A synthetic with the for-

mula 2-diethylaminoethyl-1-phenyl-cyclopentane carb-
oxylate hydrochloride (Fig. 17). It is manufactured
by Geigy Pharmaceuticals and is available in red tablets of 12½ mg. and orange tablets of 50 mg. size. It
is of value as a muscle relaxant among patients who
can tolerate it, but gastric and cerebral circulatory
reactions of giddiness, dizziness and nausea prevent
its use in arteriosclerotic and older idiopathic cases
(Sciarra, Carter and Merritt, 1949).

Tolserol (Mephenesin, Myanesin). This is a synthetic with the structural formula of 3-ortholoxy-1,2-
propanediol (Fig. 17). It is marketed by E. R. Squibb
& Sons in white tablets of 250 and 500 mg. size (Plate
1) and also in parenteral solution of 50 and 100 cc.
ampules, each cc. containing 20 mg. The drug holds
tremendous pharmacologic interest, but actually has
little practical value in parkinsonism. The parenteral
solution is occasionally employed to advantage in relaxing contractured muscles prior to physiotherapy,
but the tablets have limited use, because 12 to 20 per
day are required for effective therapy and the side
reactions of nausea and weakness prove disturbing to
the patients (Schlesinger, 1948; Hunter, 1948).

Diparcol. This synthetic has the structural formula
of diethylamino,2,ethyl-N-dibenzoparathiazine hydrochloride. It was originally manufactured by the
Rhone Chemical Society of Paris, and was distributed
for investigational purposes by Merck & Company in
62.5 and 250 mg. white tablets, until discontinued
three years ago. More recently it has been distributed
in this country through Poulenc, Ltd., of Montreal,
Canada. It is a powerful muscle relaxant with curare-
like effects (Duff, 1949), but disturbing side reactions
limit its use to postencephalitic patients, who possess

tremendous tolerance for all types of drugs. It has little if any action against tremor, nor any action as a cerebral stimulant; hence, it usually has to be combined with other drugs.

Parsidol (Lysivane, W483). This synthetic compound is closely related in chemical structure to Diparcol. It bears the formula of diethylamino-propyl-N-dibenzoparathiazine hydrochloride. It was originally manufactured by Rhone Chemical Society of Paris, and distributed in this country through Poulenc, Ltd., of Montreal, but is now manufactured by Warner-Chilcott Laboratories. It comes in 10 and 50 mg. scored white tablets and is administered in 20 mg. doses q.i.d. to older patients and 50 mg. to younger patients. It is reported (Palmer and Gallagher, 1950) to be less toxic than Diparcol and causes no dryness or blurred vision. Timberlake and Schwab (1952) report 19 to 53 per cent successes.

Pipanol (trihexyphenidyl). This synthetic compound is chemically identical with Artane. It is manufactured by Winthrop-Stearns, Inc. The vehicle in which the tablet is prepared and the method of preparation are perhaps different from that of Artane, since most of the patients reject Pipanol and favor the latter drug. Pipanol is marketed in 2 mg. white tablets only.

Pagitane (cycrimine, Compound #08958). This synthetic product is closely related in structure and action to Artane and bears the formula—1-hydroxy-1-phenyl-1-cyclohexyl-3-piperidino propane hydrochloride (Fig. 17). It is produced by Eli Lilly & Co., in $1\frac{1}{4}$ and $2\frac{1}{2}$ mg. tablets (Plate 1). It had been studied under the name "Compound 08958," but recently the name

Pagitane was applied to the product and it has been released to the trade. It is a gentle preparation, reduces rigidity and tremor and acts as a cerebral stimulant. It is effective against oculogyria. The side reactions of dryness of the mouth and blurring of vision are less than with Artane. It is safe to use in all types of parkinsonism. It is administered in the smaller size tablet b.i.d. to older patients and in 2½ mg. size q.i.d. to younger patients. Pagitane is an excellent addition to the armamentarium. It especially fills the need for a dependable preparation when other drugs begin to wear off in effects (Magee and DeJong, 1953; Zier and Doshay, to be published). It may be used as the drug of choice in commencing treatment with a new patient.

Cogentin (benztropine sulfonate, MK-02). This drug has just been approved by the Food and Drug Administration and is expected to be on the market shortly. It has the structural formula of tropine benzohydryl ether methane sulfonate (Fig. 17). It is produced by Sharp and Dohme Division of Merck & Company in 1 mg. and 2 mg. white tablets (Plate 1). It is a synthetic that combines the active radicles of atropine and Benadryl. It is a most powerful muscle relaxant, with a curare-like action. It has a cumulative effect which is of advantage in an illness such as parkinsonism, where several drugs are often required to control different symptoms. MK-02 needs to be taken only once a day on retiring. MK-02 has no cerebral stimulating action, hence needs Artane, Pagitane, or Dexedrine to supplement it. It is administered in 1 mg. doses to older patients upon retiring, and in 2, 3 or 4 mg. doses to younger patients. It counteracts spasm and cramps of the legs and toes and severe grades of rigidity and contracture, better than any drug currently available for parkinsonism (Doshay, 1952). Moreover, because of the Benadryl component in its formula, it allays excitement, tension and restlessness, controls the major form of tremor and brings sleep to insomnic patients in 37 per cent of cases (Doshay, 1953). Unlike Benadryl, however, it does not cause drowsiness, mental fogginess or "dopiness" during the day. The usual side effects are dryness of the mouth and blurred vision, and an occasional skin rash in allergic patients. Upon stopping the drug or reduction of the dosage, the rash disappears.

Synthetic Antihistaminics

Thephorin (*phenindamine*). This is a synthetic antihistaminic that has come into considerable use in parkinsonism. It has the formula, 2-methyl-9-phenyl-2.3.4.9 tetrahydro-1-pyridindene hydrogen tartrate (Fig. 17). It is marketed by Hoffmann-LaRoche Company in 25 mg. yellow tablets (Plate 1). It has some muscle relaxant action and provides a feeling of well-being to the patient, but has slight, if any, effect on tremor. It is administered two or three times a day and has to be employed along with other drugs, since alone it does not possess sufficient potency. It causes minimal side reactions and shows none of the somnolence and mental fogginess that feature the intake of Benadryl (Effron and Denker, 1950).

Benadryl (*diphenhydramine*). The structural formula of this synthetic antihistaminic is: D-dimethyl amino ethyl benzohydryl ether hydrochloride (Fig. 17). It is manufactured by Parke Davis Company in 25 mg. red and white capsules, and 50 mg. red capsules. It is one of our best current drugs for the control of

tremor, tension and excitement, and is helpful to patients who suffer from insomnia (Ryan and Wood,
1949). It is generally employed in 50 mg. doses two
to four times a day. However, the side reactions of
somnolence and mental fogginess prove disturbing to
some of the older patients, in whom it should be employed at bed-time only (Doshay, 1951). The drug
causes a trace of dryness and mydriasis, and has no
action against rigidity.

Synthetic Cerebral Stimulants

Dexedrine. This synthetic is the dextrorotary iso-
mer of Benzedrine and has a stronger central stimulating action and less of the peripheral pressor action.
Its structural formula appears in Figure 17. It is manufactured by Smith, Kline & French Laboratories in
the form of heart-shaped, peach-colored, scored tablets,
each containing 5 mg. of the active ingredient (Plate
1). It is administered in half tablets once or twice a
day to older patients, and in half or full tablets two to
six times a day to younger patients, depending upon
the need. Stronger doses are employed against narcolepsy and lesser amounts to counteract akinesia, lethargy, tiredness and weakness. Dexedrine also comes
in the form of a 15 mg. Spansule, which has a delayed
and long-lasting effect of 6 to 16 hours in different
patients. In arteriosclerotic cases, one Spansule in
the morning is sufficient. For younger patients, two
to four a day may be employed.

Benzedrine (amphetamine). This is a sympatho-
mimetic synthetic amine, with pressor activity, medullary respiratory stimulation and *almost specific cerebral stimulation of unexplainable dynamics.* It is
manufactured by Smith, Kline & French Laboratories

in heart-shaped, pink colored, scored tablets, each containing 10 mg. of the active ingredient. It is employed in half or full tablets, two or four times a day, and even in higher dosage for narcolepsy. It is used for the same indications as Dexedrine, except that it has stronger "adrenergic" actions. It is ten times as strong as caffeine in overcoming fatigue and lasts five times as long. It should be avoided in arteriosclerotic patients, because of the rise in blood pressure and tachycardia. For them, preference should be given to Dexedrine.

Other Drugs

Genoscopolamine (aminoxide of homatropine) is sometimes employed as a substitute for hyoscine, when patients cannot tolerate the disturbing side effects of the latter drug. It comes in tiny blue tablets, each containing 0.5 mg. of the active ingredient. Patients take as many as six to ten tablets a day. The side reactions and effects are minimal. *Barbiturates* in small dosage upon retiring serve to allay excitement and sleeplessness among some patients and indirectly afford a measure of relief from tremor. However, they should be avoided as a regular practice in parkinsonism, because they linger in the body, leave the patient "dopey" for 18 to 24 hours and retard motor activity. *Bromides* in small amounts may be combined with *tincture hyoscyamus* or *tincture stramonium* and sometimes prove helpful to elderly patients in alleviating tension and tremor. *Caffeine,* in the form of strong coffee or tablets, has little value in parkinsonism, because of the fleeting nature of the effects. *Curare* holds great historic and pharmacologic interest, but is of no practical value in the treatment of parkinsonism.

Vitamins, in the form of 100 mg. thiamin chloride tablets b.i.d., are employed to good advantage in cases with loss of appetite or difficulty in swallowing. Also, B_{12} injections, 100 mcg. t.i.w., or 1000 mcg. weekly, can be added temporarily for patients weakened by an operation or debilitated. *Hormones* are rarely required, except in menopause cases where a tablet of Benzestrol, 2 mg., may be given q.a.m. *Alcohol,* in moderate dosage, proves relaxing to some patients and should not be prohibited, especially if benefit is derived in lessened tremor, better appetite, etc. *Histamine* injections and infusions obtained careful study in the past and were found to be of little value in parkinsonism. *Parenteral therapy* in general should be avoided in this chronic progressive ailment, especially since oral remedies are available, that are just as good or better.

THE RESULTS

The results of therapy in parkinsonism cannot be stated with precision, because we still lack the necessary tools for the exact measurement of rigidity and tremor. Opinions based on clinical impressions alone are often misleading and explain the fact that widely differing reports are produced by observers studying the same compound, especially if a small series of cases is employed, or a faulty sampling. Generally speaking, however, a trained observer who has sufficient time for careful observation of a drug in a large enough sampling of cases, covering all three types of Parkinson patients, can arrive at a good clinical approximation of its merits and deficiencies.

On such basis, one can list the results of the commonly used Parkinson drugs, with plus signs representing approximate values:

1. *Drugs that combat rigidity*
   a. MK-02 ++++
   b. Atropine +++
   c. Artane ++
   d. Pagitane ++
   e. Thephorin +
   f. Rabellon +
   g. Vinobel +
   h. Panparnit +

2. *Drugs for use against tremor*
   a. Hyoscine ++++
   b. Benadryl +++
   c. Stramonium ++
   d. Artane +
   e. MK-02 +
   f. Pagitane +

3. *Drugs against akinesia and lethargy*
   a. Dexedrine +++
   b. Benzedrine ++
   c. Artane ++
   d. Pagitane ++

4. *Drugs for use against oculogyria*
   a. Artane +++
   b. Atropine ++
   c. Bellabulgara +
   d. Hyoscine +
   e. Rabellon +
   f. Benzedrine +

The results of therapy in parkinsonism will depend not only upon the intrinsic qualities of the drugs, but upon how well they are combined with other drugs to combat the presenting symptoms, upon the stage of illness, and upon the tolerance of the patient.

The results will also to some extent depend upon the personality of the patient, the background, the home environment, emotional security, etc. For example, one little woman of 65, with bilateral major tremor and considerable rigidity, travels and moves about as much as possible, busies herself with chores at home and is always looking at the brighter side of life. Another woman of similar age with even less tremor and rigidity spends all her time bemoaning her fate and worrying about the day when she will be completely disabled. The personality enters as a factor in the treatment here, as it does in multiple sclerosis, epilepsy, syphilis, etc.

Finally, it must be realized that drugs have little meaning in a chronic progressive illness such as parkinsonism, unless combined with continuous medical supervision, psychotherapy and physiotherapy. The patient should be seen by his doctor at regular intervals, since drugs tend to wear off in effects and others have to be substituted or added. Side reactions have to be noted and attended to. New drugs are appearing in rapid stride and the patient should receive the benefit of those most suited to him.

Psychotherapy must be made an integral part of the treatment, since it can very materially affect the results and outlook. Supportive psychotherapy should be administered during each visit, to reassure the patient and to maintain his spirited co-operation.

Physiotherapy should be administered two or three times a week, until the doctor is satisfied that there is a minimum of contracture, postural abnormality, or limitation of motion at any joints of the body. Some patients require no outside physiotherapy, since for them regular exercises at home are sufficient. "An ounce of prevention is worth a ton of cure." This particularly applies here, because Parkinson patients do not tolerate splints, braces, or plaster jackets to counteract deformities. Hence the time to prevent contracture and deformity is never too early. A full discussion of physiotherapy will appear in the chapter under that heading.

SIDE REACTIONS AND THEIR MANAGEMENT

The treatment of parkinsonism is not without difficulties. There are times when side reactions from
drugs may be almost, if not more, disturbing to the
patient than the illness itself.

Dryness of the Mouth. Almost all anti-Parkinson
drugs, and especially the belladonna preparations,
cause some dryness of the mouth. When of moderate
proportions, the patient should be advised to keep the
mouth moistened with water, to chew gum, or to use
hard lemon, lime, or cherry candies. Some drugs are
best spaced apart, or taken after meals to avoid dryness, or broken in splinters and taken q.2 h. In instances where the patient's throat, lips and tongue
become so parched that he has difficulty in swallowing,
loses weight and his speech becomes inarticulate, the
offending preparation must be discontinued in favor
of a more suitable drug. *Pilocarpine* is incapable of
counteracting the effects of atropine, hence cannot
prevent dryness of the mouth. Moreover, it causes
gastric and other reactions and is of little practical
value in this illness.

Blurring of Vision. Like dryness of the mouth, this
occurs to some degree in almost every patient under
anti-Parkinson therapy. It, however, offers less of a
challenge to treatment, since it can be overcome by
the use of suitable glasses or the instillation of *DFP*.
The latter, in a solution of 0.05 per cent, if instilled
one drop in each eye once a week, is powerful enough
to prevent or control blurring of vision caused by
atropine.

Nausea and Vomiting. Nausea is reported by 2 to

5 per cent of treated Parkinson patients. It is usually due to excessive dryness of the throat, to an incidental gastric upset, or hypersensitiveness in the patient. Vomiting, on the other hand, is rarely encountered except when atropine is employed in high dosage. While a complaint of nausea is not of special significance, vomiting regularly demands close attention, since it could be a danger signal of toxicity.

Cerebral Reactions. Complaints of mental confusion, "fogginess" and "dizziness" are uncommon in young patients, but appear frequently among the arteriosclerotic patients, particularly if a medication lowers the blood pressure and disturbs the cerebral circulation. Care should be exercised in the choice of drugs and the amounts prescribed to elderly patients.

Other Reactions. *Weakness* is occasionally attributed by patients to a particular drug when actually it is not a reaction to therapy, but part of the illness. *Bladder hesitancy* occurs in mild form with many of the belladonna preparations, but is rarely a problem unless prostatic hypertrophy exists. *Tachycardia* appears as a complaint only if drugs with strong parasympatholytic effects are employed or in highly nervous patients.

Despite all that has been said about side reactions, it can be safely stated that although a number of preparations prove disturbing to some patients from time to time, they are rarely serious. The worst that happens is that the patient becomes disgruntled, discontinues his medication and perhaps stops visiting his doctor. Even so, since treatment is not practiced for the mere sake of going through motions, but to provide relief and comfort to the patient, it must be obvious that failing to do so is not good therapy. Hence, more than ordinary care in the selection of drugs and the size of the dose will help prevent unpleasant reactions for the patient and disappointments for the doctor.

THE TREATMENT PROGRAM

Some patients require no more than one drug to keep them comfortable. This often depends upon the type of drug employed and the severity of the symptoms. Artane and Pagitane, for example, possess an action against all the cardinal symptoms of parkinsonism. However, even so-called best drugs frequently demand combination with other preparations in order to achieve maximum results. Thus, Artane in 30 to 40 per cent of cases requires the addition of hyoscine or Benadryl for the control of severe tremor, and atropine or MK-02 to counteract advanced grades of rigidity, spasm and contracture.

Still other drugs are remarkably good for the control of one symptom, but are not much good in other respects. Thus, hyoscine is an excellent drug for the control of tremor, but it has little or no action against rigidity. It is often necessary, therefore, to explore until one finds the most suitable combination of drugs that will keep the patient active and comfortable. Some patients thrive on as many as four or five preparations and are always inquiring about a new drug to be added. It is perhaps good psychotherapy to keep such patients occupied with harmless drug routines. Others resent too many drugs, especially if these involve a time-consuming program. For them, twice-a-day therapy should be arranged.

In planning treatment with a new patient, it is always desirable to inquire into past anti-Parkinson remedies, their effects and reactions. Figure 11 will render it easy for the patient to identify any medication previously employed, so that poorly-tolerated preparations may be avoided.

What also has to be taken into consideration is the age, weight, type of illness and disposition of the patient. As a rule, the older the patient, the less he is able to tolerate large doses of drugs. An obese patient is generally of easier disposition and has greater tolerance for drugs than a thin individual. Postencephalitic patients possess tremendous tolerance for every kind of drug (Doshay, 1942), whereas arteriosclerotic patients are generally sensitive to drug therapy. Again, a patient severely depressed by disabilities, economic problems and the future outlook is poor material for therapy, regardless of what drugs are employed. In such event, only traces of medication should be administered in order to obviate needless complaints of reactions, and the therapy must rest heavily on psychotherapy.

Thus, while a knowledge of the action of each drug is important, it is equally important to employ good judgment when combining the individual drugs, so as to effectively counteract all the presenting symptoms. For example, in the treatment of a young patient with rigidity and akinesia, one could combine atropine and Benzedrine, and for rigidity and tremor, atropine and hyoscine. For a middle-aged patient under similar conditions, one could combine Artane and Dexedrine, or Artane and hyoscine. For an elderly patient, one could use smaller doses of the same.

Aside from the cardinal symptoms, other symptoms require attention from time to time. *Oculogyria* is safely controlled by Artane, atropine, hyoscine, or Benzedrine. *Diplopia, weakness of ocular convergence* and *strabismus* rarely pose a problem for therapy, and the first two are helped by antispasmodics. *Sialorrhea* is regularly checked by the belladonna preparations, acting as parasympatholytic drugs. *Torticollis, dystonic* and *myoclonic movements* are favorably acted upon by belladonna and its congeners, especially 0.5 per cent atropine solution, Artane and MK-02. *Lethargy* is regularly associated with sluggishness and akinesia, so that cerebral stimulants that counteract akinesia likewise exert an action against lethargy. *Speech disorders* may be improved by deep breathing exercises and by impressing the patient to employ his lips more effectively during articulation.

Fixed facies may be improved to some degree by strong relaxants, by persistent exercise of the facial muscles and by frequent massage of the face with cream or cocoa butter. *Poor body balance* can sometimes be corrected remarkably by physiotherapy and by teaching the patient to mobilize *rapid* trunk movements forward, backward and sideways. The patient is to use a wide base in standing or walking to insure greater stability. *Contractures* that bring about flexion of the trunk and deformities of the fingers and limbs cannot be prevented in all cases, but strong muscle relaxants and regular massage and exercise can keep them under safe control for many years and in some cases they can be prevented altogether. It would do well for every patient to remember that "just as running water never freezes, so moving muscles do not freeze, shrink, or ache."

Mental symptoms are primarily due to excessive medication, to depression arising from advanced disability, or to discouragements emanating from the environment, such as the loss of employment, family conflict, etc. The first of the causes is readily helped by reducing or discontinuing the offending medication. The second requires special Parkinson convalescent homes. The third type may require *shock therapy* or psychotherapeutic guidance.

THE FUTURE OUTLOOK

Much progress has been made in the understanding and treatment of parkinsonism during the past decade, but much more remains to be done. For many patients, the future has been brightened by the advent of synthetic remedies and the steady addition of useful drugs to the armamentarium. For others, the future means disability, infirmity, invalidism and no place to go for care. We are hopefully looking to the day when, through empirical fortune or persistent exploration, more effective drugs may be discovered for parkinsonism that will afford complete relief from tremor and rigidity and be free of the disturbing side reactions of current preparations.

We stand in need of a clearer understanding from the pathologist and neurophysiologist as to the origin and pathways of tremor and rigidity, so that the neurosurgeon may know where and what to cut in order to afford relief to the patient, and so that pharmaceutical research workers may be able to prepare suitable animal subjects for the testing of prospective Parkinson compounds. We need precise instruments for the measurement of changes produced in patients by drugs and other therapies. We are in immediate need of special Parkinson convalescent homes to provide care and treatment to the advanced and disabled patients who, through misfortune or depression now terminate in State Hospitals where they do not belong.

BIBLIOGRAPHY

1. Adams, F. M., and P. L. Hays: Atropine treatment of parkinsonian syndrome. J. Oklahoma M. A., 26: 443, 1933.

2. Alcock, S., and E. A. Carmichael: Treatment of parkinsonism with Bulgarian belladonna. Quart. J. Med., 7:565, 1938.

3. Corbin, K. B.: Trihexyhphenidyl (artane, piperidine compound) in treatment of parkinsonism. J. A. M. A., 141:377, 1949.

4. Doshay, L. J.: Moderate-dosage atropine treatment of the Parkinson syndrome. New York J. Med., 42: 1066, 1942.

5. ——: Recent trends in the treatment of parkinsonism. M. Rec., 160:339, 1947.

6. ——, and Constable, K.: Artane therapy for parkinsonism. J. A. M. A., 140:1317, 1949.

7. ——: Newer drugs in the treatment of parkinsonism. Neurology, 1:68, 1951.

8. ——, et al.: Preliminary study of a new antiparkinson agent. Neurology, 2:233, 1952.

9. ——, and A. Zier: Minor and major tremor in parkinsonism. The outcomes in 544 treated cases. Neurology, 3:360, 1953.

10. ——: Parkinsonism (Postencephalitic, Idiopathic and Arteriosclerotic). Current Therapy. W. B. Saunders, Philadelphia, 1953, p. 652.

11. ——: The Therapy of Parkinsonism. M. Clin. North America. Saunders, Philadelphia, 1953, p. 1511.

12. ——: Five-year follow-up of Artane treatment; the outcome of 461 cases of parkinsonism. J. A. M. A., (in process of publication).

13. Dow, R. S., and H. Rosenbaum: The treatment of parkinsonism with Artane. Northwest Med., 48:699, 1949.

14. Duff, R. S.: Use of Diparcol in parkinsonism. Brit. M. J., 1:613, 1949.
15. Effron, A. S., and P. G. Denker: Antispasmodic drugs in Parkinson's disease. J. A. M. A., 144:5, 1950.
16. Ellenbogen, B. K.: Artane in the treatment of parkinsonism. Lancet, 1:1034, 1950.
17. Epidemic Encephalitis, Third Report of the Matheson Commission, Vol. 53. New York, Columbia University Press, 1939, p. 65.
18. Hill, D.: Bulgarian treatment of postencephalitic parkinsonism. Lancet, 2:1048, 1938.
19. Hunter, A. R., and J. M. Waterfall: Myanesin in hyperkinetic states. Lancet, 1:366, 1948.
20. Kleeman, A.: Die chronische encephalitis und ihre behandlung. Med. Woch. f. Wurtenberg, 99:1, 1929.
21. Magee, K. R., and R. N. De Jong: Antispasmodic Compound 08958 in treatment of paralysisagitans. J. A. M. A., 153:715, 1953.
22. Neal, J. B.: Recent advances in treatment of epidemic encephalitis. New York J. Med., 34:707, 1934.
23. ———, and S. M. Dillenberg: Belladonna and other forms of medication. New York J. Med., 40:1300, 1940.
24. Palmer, H., and D. J. A. Gallagher: Lysivane therapy for parkinsonism. Brit. M. J., 2:558, 1950.
25. Phillips, J., E. Montuschi, and J. Sharkey: Artane in the treatment of parkinsonism. Lancet, 1:1131, 1950.
26. Price, J. C., and H. H. Meritt: Bulgarian belladonna and alkaloids of U.S.P. belladonna. J. A. M. A., 117:335, 1941.
27. Römer, C.: Zur Atropinbehandlung der encephalitische Folgezustande. Ztschr. f. d. ges. Neur. & Psych., 132: 724, 1931.
28. Ryan, G. M. S., and J. S. Wood: Benadryl in the treatment of parkinsonism. Results of forty cases. Lancet, 1:258, 1949.
29. Schlesinger, E. B., A. L. Drew, and B. Wood: Clinical studies in the use of Myanesin. Am. J. Med., 4:365, 1948.
30. Sciarra, D., S. Carter, and H. H. Meritt: Panparnit in the treatment of diseases of the basal ganglions. J. A. M. A., 141:1226, 1949.

102   Drug Therapy

31. Shapiro, S. K.: Drug therapy in parkinsonism. Minnesota Med., **35**:1031, 1952.
32. Sollman, T.: A Manual of Pharmacology. Philadelphia, W. B. Saunders Co., 1936, p. 379.
33. Timberlake, W. H., and R. S. Schwab: Experimental preparation W-483 in the treatment of Parkinson's disease. New England J. Med., **247**:98, 1952.
34. Vollmer, H.: The Bulgarian treatment of postencephalitic parkinsonism. J. Mt. Sinai Hosp., **6**:93, 1939.
35. von Wetzleben, H. D.: Methods of Treatment in Postencephalitic Parkinsonism. New York, Grune & Stratton, 1942, p. 113.
36. Zier, A., and L. J. Doshay: Treatment of parkinsonism with Pagitane. Results in 142 cases. (To be published.)

7

PHYSICAL THERAPY

WILLIAM BENHAM SNOW, M.D.

THE Parkinson syndrome represents a group of symptoms which usually tend to progress in extent and severity. Parkinsonism of any extent, however, represents a disability in which rehabilitation technics are indicated and considerable amelioration of the symptoms can be effected.

Patients with parkinsonism are prone to drift into loneliness, with inner feelings of physical frustration and community rejection. Social contacts become difficult and patients develop a marked lack of motivation. They tend to become dejected, depressed and inactive, with increasing tissue functional degeneration, due to lack of mobility. With the ageing process, degenerative changes set in, such as arthritis, the progress of which is apt to increase due to lack of exercise of the joints, so necessary to retention of normal joint circulation and function. The increasing rigidity of muscles and the forced positioning of the joints result in strain and fatigue. Disuse and injury of muscle substance lead to chronic myofibrositis and restriction of muscle length. Thereby, severe and painful contractures often result at the fingers, wrists, toes, ankles, elbows, knees, shoulders and hips. Contracture of the thigh adductors is a common source of great pain and discomfort. The shortened muscles tend to twist the joints out of shape and lead to deformities of varying degree.

Since the myofibrositis, contractures and deformities can be greatly lessened by consistent and intensive therapy, it must be realized that the syndrome of parkinsonism represents a challenge to those interested in rehabilitation. The patients can do much for themselves, but discouragements, disabilities and discomforts demand outside help.

TOTAL NEEDS OF THE PATIENT

The needs are psychological and physical. The aims of physical medicine and rehabilitation in parkinsonism must be geared toward these needs. Even so, physical medicine and rehabilitation technics are but part of the broader program that should be made available to every patient, and they should be synchronized with the other modalities of treatment. All those who have contact with the patient, family, friends, co-workers, doctors and therapists, should aim to bolster the spirits and physical well-being of the patient, so that he may continue functioning for many years, to the maximum satisfaction of himself and those close to him.

Neither nature nor medication can overcome the pathology, but the altered physiological reactions can be sufficiently modified or reversed by therapy, so as to permit the patient to remain productive and cheerful, despite his disability. Under suitable guidance and aid, the patient can learn to have faith in the future and to adjust to his disability. In this age when

medical matters are so widely disclosed to the lay pub-
lic, often with little judgment and tact, patients soon
acquire the information that they are suffering from a
progressive malady.   For this reason, there comes a
time, early or late, when the patient's confidence is
best gained by presenting the truth to him, tempered
with kindness, reassurance and hopefulness.

Physical Assistance

The Parkinson tremor is of the resting type and is
amenable to diminution by voluntary movement
(Bach, 1950; Steiglitz, 1949).   It can be lessened in
extent if the mind of the patient is diverted toward
activity, thereby less attention comes to be paid to
the tremor by the patient and those about him.

The rigidity is due to an overactivity of antagonists,
both flexion and extension.   However, since this is an
illness where flexion contractures of wrists, elbows,
knees, neck and trunk are more dominant, it is com-
batted by exercise activities that increase extension at
the flexed joints.   Massage proves helpful in some of
these situations.

The slowness of voluntary motion in response to
commands can be counteracted by definitive drilling
of various kinds.

The atrophy of disuse and contractures due to physiological adaptive shortening can be offset by well
planned, progressive resistive exercise procedures in
occupational therapy and physical therapy.

The shuffling, unsteady, cumbersome gait can be
corrected by critical walking training and certain
tricks which the therapist can effectively employ in
his technics.   Improved general body co-ordination,
such as getting out of a chair, getting in and out of

bed, etc., can be achieved by carefully conceived and motivated drilling.

Activities of Daily Living

The clumsiness and ineptness of performing functions necessary to everyday existence, such as details of dressing, eating, grooming, toilet activities and writing, all may be improved if properly worked upon (Buchwald, 1952). Experience has shown that some patients can be rehabilitated for earning activities, often returning to work or developing new activities or hobbies within their special spheres of accomplishment. Except in the few advanced cases where mental function has actually been impaired by cerebral circulatory impoverishment, these individuals can be motivated from their disconsolate semi-lethargy and helped to regain some joy in living.

Importance of Therapeutic Interest

The rehabilitation is not a matter of prescribing physical and occupational therapy procedures. It can only be accomplished through the personal interest of those carrying out the program and through flexibility in the arrangement of rehabilitation procedures *per se,* motivated by this personal interest. Patients will respond favorably to such psychological approach and, even if despondent and possessed of skeptical and depressed feelings, will evidence a desire to apply themselves to the therapeutic program. Moreover, the change in attitude and interest of the patient in responding to the treatment cannot fail to find reflection in enthusiastic reactions on the part of the family, which is essential to the success of the treatment regime.

THE PHYSICAL PROGRAM

At this point we shall attempt to describe the technics generally employed in occupational and physical therapy. This cannot, however, fully present the integration necessary for effective accomplishment. It will be more logical if we consider the physiological problems, and then bring the technical treatment in line to meet the needs.

For improving the gait, one could simply say that gait training is indicated and be correct. However, gait training is a complicated procedure and the elements of faulty gait differ from one phase of the disease to another. Unless the integers which are disturbed and which add up to a good walking pattern are reviewed independently, improved walking will not result. There are weak muscles which need strengthening. There are shortened structures which need stretching. There are rigid components and frozen muscular attitudes which may have to be loosened, stretched and warmed up before the patient can even begin to function.

The normal reciprocal pattern of motion will have to be reinforced. The use of bicycle actions and the altered rhythmic movements of upper and lower extremities must be worked upon. Often rolling, crawling and creeping activities will assist in attaining reciprocity. Trunk and spinal rigidity may be released by active calisthenics. Music can do much to enhance the development of rhythmic activities.

Posture Correction

Regular walking exercises should be carried out. Accent on the heel-stepping gait will do much to slow down the tendency to propulsion. An obstacle course to make shuffling impossible and to increase the motivation toward flexion of the hips is very helpful. This can be accomplished by the use of irregularly placed lumber in the path of the patient.

While the patient is in the occupational therapy shop he should be kept moving and not placed on static activities. During each session the patient should have a well planned, diversified group of activities.

Other exercises that enter into improved walking and daily utilitarian needs are those which have to do with improving muscular co-ordination. Among the physical therapy procedures, the precision exercise routine of Frenkel is most desirable for some patients (Coulter, 1936). Frenkel exercises are based upon the principle that movements are carried out and directed from pictured movements which occur at the cerebral level. To re-educate a person in co-ordinated movement, training is carried out step by step as though the individual were entirely unaccustomed to carrying out basic movements. New patterns for co-ordination are built up in this way. The speed of performance occurs as increased facility progresses. Frenkel has described a complete system of these exercises.

Massage

In physical therapy, massage is sometimes given patients because it is pleasing to them. When muscles are immobilized as is the case in this disease, certainly manipulation of them feels good and actually improves the circulatory status of the muscles (Bierman and Licht, 1952). It is probably better, however, to reserve the skilled massage therapy for cases that develop myofibrositic changes with painful symptoms. These situations respond even better to heat applications, moist or dry, instituted prior to the massage.

Muscle Stretching

The immobilized, stiffened, or rigid muscles of parkinsonism are best treated by muscle stretching. This should be *forceful,* but only within physiological joint planes and with a knowledge of safe range of motion of each restricted joint. A vigorous muscle stretching program is often uncomfortable, and in the first days of treatment may not be particularly enjoyable to the patient. However, the relief in flexibility afforded the patient by such stretching of muscles and fascia will make the patient look forward to more of such treatments. Often after a period of inactivity, stretching of the patient by a member of his family will start him off on a more relaxed and improved postural movement. The training of a suitable member of the family in the proper use of stretching exercises can prove of material assistance in the treatment program.

Progressive Resistive Exercise

As physiological relaxation of antagonists occurs with voluntary activity of a muscle, and as this relaxation is proportionate in degree to the intensity of the muscular effort, progressive resistive exercises promote muscular relaxation (Watkins and DeLorme, 1951). They likewise help in strengthening the weak muscles which, due to inactivity, have lost reserve functional strength.

Occupational Therapy

In occupational therapy, many functional activities

can be utilized to build up the intrinsic quality of muscles and to improve co-ordination (Bach, 1950, Dunton, 1950).

Woodwork. Woodworking offers large motions of both upper extremities for maintaining voluntary motion. Sanding with a two-handed sander, on a level or an incline, and sawing with a ripsaw encourage gross shoulder and elbow motion and enhance hand grasp. The use of the coping saw gives forearm function, smaller muscle activities and finer co-ordination and control. Filing with a two-handed file has a utility similar to the two-handed sander, but in addition may be used for more co-ordinated two-joint functions.

Weaving. This makes use of perpendicular braid weave looms which utilize heavy material, enhance gross shoulder and elbow activities. The floor loom calls into action the co-ordinated use of both upper and lower extremities, exercising all joints in a multiplicity of movements. Positioning of the patient close to or far from the loom, high or low, modifies the range of lower extremity function. The loom may be weighted to add resistance to the effort required.

The manually operated *printing press* gives gross shoulder activities in forcing the handle down and requires co-ordination of both hands in placing and removing the paper. Critical posturing of the patient during the operation of the press is to be done. Setting type requires finer co-ordination and utilizes fingers and thumb in opposition.

Writing. The patient is placed before a blackboard and asked to draw lines as straight, horizontal, or perpendicular, to draw geometric figures, and make circles and the like. One starts with gross shoulder motions. It is interesting to watch the patient master first the horizontal line, the circle, and later the perpendicular line, progressing from tremorous irregular movements to evenly drawn, straight lines. Placement of the chalk improves and the hand grows steadier as skill progresses. The amount of the board available for use of the patient is restricted in accordance with manifest improvement. The use of the fountain pen should be encouraged, particularly in writing the signature, because it is often an economic need and also because it harbors psychological value.

Activities of Daily Living. The patient is tested and the number of things that he cannot accomplish on his own are listed. He is then put through a training that will successively reduce these to an inconsequential minimum.

Group Games of Low Organization. When a number of patients can be brought together, recreational group games of low organization, not requiring keen skill or competition, are of great help in motivating them to greater activity and emotional expressiveness (Morgan, 1948). Patients under such routines look forward with anticipation to these group play periods.

THE HOME PROGRAM

Unless a Parkinson patient is treated within a resident institution, the definitive rehabilitation regime of occupational therapy, physical therapy, or recreation will generally fail of its aim, unless reinforced by a home program. The ambulatory patient needs the home program to carry over the motivation and other benefits gained during his out-patient visits.

The success of the home program will, of course, depend upon all the multiple factors which are cumulatively present in any individual patient's home. The greatest single factor is intelligent co-operation from other members of the household. On the diligence and application of these in carrying out a planned regime will depend any hope of a satisfactory result. If good rapport can be established within the home, the clinical program will be immensely more effective than any gain that could be achieved through out-patient therapy alone. Suggestions for such a program might be:

Gardening Activities. These could include the use of a hoe for weeding and mounding soil; the raking of leaves; mowing the lawn; sprinkling; pruning with saw or pruning shears; crawling activities necessary to planting and weeding, etc.

Walking. Patients should be reminded not to sit motionless for long periods of time. Hazards, as mentioned previously, may be utilized for prevention of shuffling.

Golfing. This can be more beneficial than walking to some patients, and there is the added incentive of gentle competition, fraternity and socialization.

Housework. The normal activities of scrubbing, sweeping, dusting, ironing and the like should be encouraged, as well as the more complicated activities associated with cooking, such as whipping potatoes, preparing vegetables, etc.

Home Exercise Games. These should preferably include shuffle board, quoits, horseshoe pitching, croquet, archery and darts, rather than long-sitting games, such as cards. Ping-pong or badminton are suited to some of the patients, but tennis and handball are generally considered too competitive, strenuous and discouraging for use as home training.

The above represents a rational physiological approach to the problems of rehabilitation presented by Parkinson patients. Proper application of these and similar methods has proven of great value in maintaining the general health and mobility of the patients and in increasing the joy and the continued service of these patients to the family and community.

BIBLIOGRAPHY

Bach: Recent Advances in Physical Medicine, Blakiston, Philadelphia, 1950, p. 6.

Bierman and Licht: Physical Medicine in General Practice, 3rd Ed., 1952, P. P. Hoeber, Inc., p. 329.

Buchwald: Physical Rehabilitation for Daily Living, 1952, McGraw-Hill Co., Inc., New York.

Coulter, Pemberton and Mock: Principles and Practice of Physical Therapy, Vol. 3, Chap. 15, pp. 30–44. Prior, Hagerstown, Md., 1936.

Dunton and Licht: Occupational Therapy—Principles and Practice, Thomas, Springfield, Ill., 1950.

Morgan: The physical reconditioning program of the army, Physical & Mental Rehab. J., 2:2, 1948.

Steiglitz: Geriatric Medicine, 2nd Ed., Saunders, Philadelphia, 1949, p. 284.

Watkins and DeLorme: Progressive Resistance Exercise, Appleton-Century-Crofts, Inc., New York, 1951.

8

PSYCHOTHERAPY

Samuel Brock, M.D.

PSYCHOTHERAPY for parkinsonism in the past depended on the conception of the underlying pathologic process. At the turn of the century, the disease was regarded as a functional one, but in the first two decades of the twentieth century and thereafter the organic basis was established pari passu with the development of understanding concerning the functions of the basal ganglia.

HISTORICAL DOCUMENTATION

A brief review of the attitude to psychotherapy in the writings of various authorities may be of interest, as revealed in some textbooks of the last four decades.

Dana (1915) notes that "patients [with paralysis agitans] are easily made better for a time by some psychical influence." He develops the theme no further.

Ramsey Hunt (1924) makes reference to the avoidance of excitement or stress and advises that the "psychotherapeutic possibilities and aspects of the case should always be considered."

Jelliffe and White (1929) comment as follows: "In the beginning of many a presenile or senile Parkinsonian syndrome, an enlightened psychotherapy may be of signal service, especially in regulating faulty emotion reactions . . . efforts that will show the patient a better philosophy of self-control are often surprisingly effective in quieting the tremor, giving rest and sleep."

Bing (1939) discusses treatment of the degenerative, arteriosclerotic and encephalitic forms of the disease but makes no specific reference to psychotherapy. Wilson (1940) and Grinker (1944) similarly make no mention of psychotherapy in parkinsonism.

Nielsen (1946) discusses psychotherapy with the statement that "constant attention and encouragement are necessary. . . . It has even been thought that the psychotherapeutic element in the treatment is the greatest single effective factor."

Wechsler (1952) speaks of "psychotherapy [as being] of benefit in most cases, even though the effect is only temporary."

PSYCHOTHERAPY AS AN AID TO BETTER ADJUSTMENT

In a strict sense, there is no directly effective psychotherapy against parkinsonism, whether of inflammatory, degenerative, arteriosclerotic or other type, since the organic disturbance is not amenable to such an approach. It is nevertheless very desirable to treat the patient by means of psychotherapy in an effort to bring about the best possible adjustment between him, his environment and the gradually crippling process. However, it should be noted that parkinsonism is not accompanied by any specific personality deviation characteristic of the disease, except for the abnormal behavior patterns of juvenile encephalitic cases noted during the 1920 decade—a rather small fraction of the total.

The individual with parkinsonism is unlike the victim of multiple sclerosis, who often shows a mild euphoria as part of his disease. The type of personality, on the other hand, which the physician is called upon to treat in parkinsonism, is determined by the individual's intrinsic make-up before he became ill. Such admixture of organic disease and personality reaction is encountered frequently in the practice of medicine, whether one is dealing with organic nervous disease, heart disease, or other visceral disease. Since the co-existence of parkinsonism and the behavior pattern present a considerable variety of reactions, it must be evident that the results of psychotherapy will vary a good deal, depending upon the patient's receptivity and responsiveness. This leaves still other variables, namely, the physician's particular aptitude for and training in psychotherapy and the attitude and the co-operation of relatives and attendants.

If one has a long experience in the handling of these patients, many instances illustrative of the patient's total reaction to his disease will come to mind.

The author recalls a man in his sixties, who had developed a moderate parkinsonism, with rigidity and tremor so characteristic of the disease. He had been a very successful banker and industrialist, who for many years had prided himself on his prowess as an equestrian, a hunter and an out-of-doors man. He had no sympathy with any of the "softer sports" or cultural activities. He was rigid, inflexible and unmoved by many attempts to interest him in other avocations. He closed all doors to entreaty and persuasion and stated that when he no longer could ride his horses and shoot from the saddle, he would commit suicide, which he did by a bullet through his head, although his disease was hardly far advanced. Here was a stubborn individual incapable of compromise or guidance, who destroyed himself, despite ample means that could have provided him with many advantages.

At the other extreme is a patient in his fifties, with a slowly progressive encephalitic parkinsonism of 15 years' duration. His muscle rigidity and festinating gait are marked; his speech is a repetitious whisper, often inaudible. He has survived the death of near relatives, continues to drive his car, visits friends, travels, takes photographs and even participates in some of the political activities of his community. He sees his physician on occasion and seeks no psychotherapeutic aid. His exuberant personality will not be quelled by obstacles imposed by the disease.

These are extreme types, representing opposite poles. In the larger middle group are the individuals who invest the disease with more or less neurotic reaction in line with their make-up prior to illness. Querulous, pathetic in their affliction, sometimes apparently without hope, yet rarely deeply depressed, these individuals do not offer a fertile soil for any special psychotherapeutic approach. Nor is the neurosis itself so disabling as to require a penetrating analysis, and very rarely, too, does such a patient have the desire or the stamina to cope with a far-flung investigation.

CHANNELING OF INTERESTS AND ACTIVITIES

Efforts should be directed toward keeping the patient's interest aroused by and channeled into activities within his intellectual and physical reach. In the older age group, this amounts to a program of restricted "rehabilitation," adapted to the advancing disability imposed by the progressing disease. Most of these measures will represent passive hobbies, rather than active ones; viz., reading or being read to, rather than painting or playing an instrument. Even so, continual encouragement and strong measures of reassurance are necessary, and *the physician must never drop the mask of optimism and hope*. To this end, one should frequently compare the patient with Mr. X. or Mrs. Y., who has the same disease in much worse form and yet manages to do thus and so.

How successfully one can inculcate a "keep-interested-and-never-say-die" attitude will depend, of course, upon the patient, the stage of the disease, the attitude of relatives and friends, and the persistence and the patience of nurses, attendants and physician. This type of program demands the education of others besides the patient, because a pessimistic attitude on the part of anyone who comes in contact with the patient may ruin the difficult psychotherapeutic regimen. The clear sensorium which most patients possess is at once a boon and a handicap. The advantage lies in being able to utilize his faculties for the development of "occupational" interests and activities of one sort or another. The disadvantage arises from the fact that often the patient is able to appraise realistically the uphill nature of the struggle and the downhill progress of his physical infirmities.

As much as possible, one should try to programatize the patient's activities in such a way as to make him feel that his day is plotted into periods of *rest, activity* and *entertainment,* rather than have him regard each day as a hit-or-miss 24 hours, without plan or schedule.

Psychotherapy must be made an integral part of the treatment, since the results are materially affected by it. A patient who becomes depressed and has misgivings as to the outcome of his illness may lose all interest in medication and physiotherapy and increase the speed of a downhill course. As part of psychotherapy, the physician must attempt to remove misconceptions about the illness and should strive to present the brighter side to the patient: viz., that parkinsonism may be kept a minor illness with proper management; that man is subject to far worse ailments, such as cancer; that the rigidity and tremor of the disease may be combated successfully by faithful exercise and treatment; that there is seldom any disabling paralysis connected with the illness, or pain; and that parkinsonism usually is unassociated with serious diseases, so that the victim may live comfortably and usefully for many years. The patient should also be advised that many newer drugs are being investigated, and some may prove to be of great value.

Thus, psychotherapy must keep up the patient's morale, and this can be accomplished only if the physician himself is well grounded in the subject and has confidence in what he is doing. Visits should be utilized by the physician not merely to check upon the symptoms but also to help the patient with his personal and related problems. The patient may wish to know whether quitting work will conserve his health and prolong his life, whether to undergo an operation, whether to use one type of laxative or another, what type of diet to employ, etc. Many such questions arise in a patient's mind, and the physician is often the only one who can provide the answer and the reassurance that will instill confidence and keep him going.

REFERENCES

Bing, Robert: Textbook of Nervous Diseases, translated and enlarged by Webb Haymaker, pp. 171, 172, 416, St. Louis, Mosby, 1939.

Dana, C. L.: Textbook of Nervous Diseases, ed. 8, p. 575, New York, Wood, 1915.

Grinker, R. R.: Neurology, ed. 3, p. 416, Springfield, Ill., Thomas, 1944.

Hunt, Ramsey: Diseases of the Nervous System, vol. 6 of Nelson's Loose Leaf Living Medicine, p. 610, New York, Nelson, 1924.

Jelliffe, S. E., and White, W. A.: Diseases of the Nervous System, ed. 5, p. 657, Philadelphia, Lea, 1929.

Nielsen, J. M.: A Textbook of Clinical Neurology, ed. 2, p. 187, New York, Hoeber, 1946.

Wechsler, I. S.: Textbook of Clinical Neurology, ed. 7, p. 576, Philadelphia, Saunders, 1952.

Wilson, S. A. K.: Neurology, vols. 1 and 2, pp. 142, 805, Baltimore, Williams & Wilkins, 1940.

9

SURGICAL THERAPY

EDWARD B. SCHLESINGER, M.D.

ONLY by rare good fortune is specific therapy for parkinsonism likely to be discovered, so long as the exact nature of tremor and rigidity remains obscure. The complexities of the problem and its intimate relationship to many unknown mechanisms of physiologic conception make it an almost unsurmountable one at our present level of knowledge.

SUMMARY OF PROCEDURES

Surgery directed at the disturbed physiologic mechanisms of Parkinson's syndrome has produced much more in the way of laboratory insights than in clinical relief. No single operative approach advanced to date has become a standard therapeutic tool. However, certain facts have been derived from the sum of the various procedures. Chief among these is that rigidity responds poorly, even in proportion to the generally imperfect effect upon tremor. Since rigidity is more complex in its central-segmental-peripheral relationships, this is not surprising. The second conclusion to be drawn from surgical experience is that the efficiency of effect upon tremor, with notable exceptions, seems to be related directly to the degree of paresis incident to the procedure.

This is not wholly an unexpected deduction. Parkinson, in his original essay of 1817, noted that an intercurrent hemiplegia arrested tremor. He likewise reported that any improvement in paralysis was reflected in a proportionate return in tremor violence. Gowers (1903), describing various forms of therapy, mentioned that stretching of the brachial plexus lessened tremor but at the price of paralysis and extensive muscle wasting. These two astute observers, if given the chance to add the present literature to their own experience, surely would conclude that destruction of the major common pathway to the periphery is still the most obvious means of influencing tremor.

On perusal of the literature, one finds that the surgical approaches, in general, reflect the anatomic and physiologic knowledge of their period. The earlier investigators utilized an attack based upon the premise of discrete centers, whose destruction should alter the pattern of abnormal activity. Later, when the hypothesis of such centers became less attractive, surgery was more and more directed at altering the bombardment to the periphery at any feasible point along the various common pathways to the segmental level. Depriving the segmental and central areas of impulses from the periphery, either by section of posterior roots or, more obliquely, the autonomics, had rapidly been proved to be useless and is without any present champion. There remain, in addition, certain procedures whose rationale is poorly understood or not consonant with present concepts, which nevertheless have shown promise or undoubted effect upon features of parkinsonism.

In spite of the great handicaps of imperfect knowledge and lack of opportunity for efficient amelioration of Parkinson mechanisms, much valuable information has been gathered by surgical investigators. Although it is tempting here to include a review of surgical treatment of extrapyramidal disease as a whole, the restriction of space and subject prevent any documentation of the literature on athetosis, dystonia and hemiballismus. The various surgical measures carried out in attempting to influence Parkinson tremor or rigidity have been gathered together and will be described briefly. For convenience, anatomic level has been chosen as a means of classification.

SURGICAL ASPECTS

I. At the Cortical Level

Extirpation of the Area of Representation of the Involved Limb in the Precentral Gyrus (Area 4)

In 1936 Aring and Fulton demonstrated that intention tremor in the monkey (secondary to cerebellar lesions) could be abolished by ablation of Areas 4 and 6. Bucy and Case (1939) removed a similar area in a patient who, after trauma to the brain, suffered from intention tremor and tremor at rest in a single upper extremity. The clinical result was and has remained excellent. Subsequently, Bucy demonstrated that ablation of Area 4 alone sufficed. Bucy (1942) carefully pointed out that his case series includes patients whose tremor followed cerebral trauma or luetic mesencephalitis. In setting up criteria for operation, he suggests that the procedure be limited to those cases with tremor of only one side of the body, in which there is reason to believe that progression of the disease is slow. In such case the resulting monoplegia is ordinarily preferable to tremor. Sachs (1942) reported that Area 6 removal alone was not effective in relieving tremor. Klemme reported a large series of cases of frank Parkinson type with excellent results after removal of frontal cortex anterior to the electrically excitable strip. His findings are difficult to interpret in view of the lack of specific information regarding his technical procedure and they have not been generally duplicated.

II. At the Level of the Basal Ganglia

A. Meyers (1942) has carried out the following procedures:

1. Extirpation of the head of the caudate nucleus.

2. Extirpation of the head of the caudate nucleus and interruption of the fibers coursing in the oral half to three fourths of the anterior limb of the internal capsules.

3. Extirpation of the head of the caudate nucleus and the oral thirds of the putamen and the globus pallidus and interruption of the fibers running in the oral fourth of the anterior limb of the internal capsule.

4. Section of the pallidofugal fibers (ansa lenticularis, fasciculus lenticularis, and "fine fibers" of Papez).

In each type of procedure he noted improvement in tremor and rigidity; greatest, however, following pallidofugal section. He considers it the simplest of the "basal ganglion type" procedures, with marked reduction or cessation of tremor and reduction in rigidity by 50 per cent or more. In a case treated by extirpation of portions of the caudate nucleus, the putamen and the globus pallidus, the unilateral tremor and severe festination were abolished. However, a monoplegia followed the operation, presumably based on damage to the blood supply of the internal capsule as it traversed the bed of the putamen.

B. Browder (1948), after exploring the various cortical and spinal approaches to the therapy of tremor, advocated section of the fibers of the anterior limb of the internal capsule, along with ablation of the adjacent anterior portion of the putamen. In his hands this procedure has proved to be the most effective means of ameliorating alternating tremor and rigidity without residual paresis. Ablation of a portion of or the total head of the caudate nucleus alone did not alter either tremor or rigidity in his series.

C. Ligation of the anterior choroidal artery. Cooper (1953) achieved a marked reduction in tremor and rigidity, after ligation of the contralateral anterior choroidal artery. Since the anterior choroidal vessel supplies the globus pallidus, he felt that the ligation played a specific part in the effected changes. An early preliminary report on subsequent cases tends to corroborate his original observation. Insufficient time has elapsed to determine the permanent value of anterior choroidal ligation. For the present, the operation is being limited to patients under 50 years of age, because of unpredictable complications in older patients.

III. At the Level of the Cerebellar Nuclei

Delmas-Marsalet and von Bogaert (1935) damaged the dentate nucleus in attempting to alleviate Parkinson tremor. Tremor became perceptibly more violent, although there was a reduction in rigidity.

IV. At the Level of the Peduncle

Walker carried out section of the anterolateral portion of the cerebral peduncle (1949), and subsequently White (1950) reported an additional case. There was definite reduction in tremor noted, even in those cases in which no hemiparesis occurred. In the absence of paresis, one must assume that the pyramidal tract was not greatly damaged. This is an excellent example of the confusing nature of data gleaned from operative reports.

V. At the Level of the Cervical Cord

A. Putnam, in 1940, reported on the effect of section of the lateral pyramidal tract. With Herz (1950), he has followed and since reported on 22 patients who have undergone this procedure. They conclude that the chance of cessation or marked reduction in tremor is of the order of 1 out of 3; of some improvement in tremor of the order of 2 out of 3. They underline the risk, however, in stating that permanent paresis occurs in 1 to 2 out of 3 cases. It is again striking that the degree of amelioration of tremor is directly proportionate to paresis and tends to lessen as motor power recovers.

The attractiveness of the procedure lies in its relative ease of performance and the avoidance of the more serious complications of cerebral ablative procedures.

B. Oliver (1949), dissatisfied with the results after section of the lateral pyramidal tract, increased the extent of the incision to include the whole of the lateral column. Postoperatively, his patients showed loss of tremor, with almost complete recovery from the induced hemiplegia but permanent hemianalgesia and hemithermanasthesia. Oliver feels that the procedure should be restricted to patients with strictly unilateral signs, even as concerns masking of the facies.

C. Ebin (1949) reported upon an extension of the Putnam lateral cordotomy to include the ventral tracts. Rigidity and tremor were strikingly alleviated after this procedure. Bilateral operation likewise afforded dramatic relief of tremor and rigidity, and the patient maintained excellent voluntary motor power and was able to walk 400 steps a day and even climb stairs.

D. Posterior Columns: Puusepp (1932) and Rizzatti and Moreno (1936) sectioned the posterior columns in an attempt to alleviate rigidity. No real clinical response of long-term benefit was obtained, and the procedure has lost vogue completely as a means of influencing rigidity.

E. Anterior Columns: Both Oldberg (1938) and Putnam (1938) failed to obtain clinical reduction in tremor following section of the anterior column of the spinal cord.

VI. At the Level of the Posterior Roots

Pollack and Davis (1930), Puusepp (1930), Foerster (1932) and others attempted to reduce rigidity by deafferentation. Section of the posterior roots had no worth-while clinical effect upon the state of the preoperative rigidity.

VII. Excision of the Superior Cervical Sympathetic Ganglion

In 1948 Gardner reported upon the results after "cerebral" sympathectomy in the treatment of Parkinson's syndrome. He noted a favorable alteration in mood, and a reduction in rigidity and improved ability to perform physical acts in a few instances. In general, he considered the procedure to be of slight value.

PRACTICAL ASPECTS OF SURGICAL MANAGEMENT

At best the Parkinson patient is not a good surgical risk. Cortical procedures such as that of Klemme and

Bucy carry a high incidence of postoperative seizures. The Parkinson brain is frequently atrophic and sclerotic and so is particularly prone to the general complications of cerebral surgery. Spinal procedures carry an impressive risk of irreversible damage following edema and vascular damage to the entire cord, and the less serious but very disabling loss of bladder and bowel control. Radicular pain, dysasthesias and postoperative pulmonary complications after cervical cordotomy are not infrequent.

Analysis of the foregoing case reports leaves one with a few specific conclusions and much confusing physiologic data. There seems to be little doubt that tremor can be influenced to some degree at any point from the highest motor representation in the premotor cortex to the level of the pyramidal tract in the cord. To conclude that interruption of the pyramidal tract is essential to this ameliorative effect is unsafe in view of Browder's demonstration of reduction of tremor after his capsular procedure without severe paresis. Also, the cases of Walker and White in which tremor was reduced without significant paresis belie the importance of pyramidal section per se. The amazing preservation of motor function claimed for the Oliver and Ebin procedures merely confuses one's traditional physiologic concepts. The exact mode of effect upon tremor and rigidity of anterior choroidal ligation is as yet not clear.

No single one of the aforementioned approaches has approached the status of a standard clinical procedure. The reasons are varied. Ablation of Area 4, for example, as Bucy clearly pointed out, must be reserved for patients with unilateral involvement, since paresis

is the price of the postoperative relief of tremor. All
of the operations which involve the cerebrum carry, in
addition to paralysis, an impressive statistical risk of
setting up epileptogenic foci. Some, such as Meyers'
battery of procedures, are very difficult to standardize
and may entail damage to adjacent structures. Certain
procedures, the immediate effects of which led to im-
moderate enthusiasm, afford no worth-while permanent relief to the patient. Some must pass into limbo
as the natural product of the worst possible means of
attaining exquisite laboratory data: human dealing
with human!

On the purely philosophical side, one may add that
surgery consists in the repair of supporting or structural elements or the extirpation of irritative, compres-
sive or invasive lesions. Where none of these conditions
applies or exists, surgery is singularly inefficient as a
therapeutic weapon. For example, reducing the number of effector volleys in a malfunctioning phasic appa-
ratus may dampen the abnormal response, but only in
proportion to a decrease in efficiency of performance.

The intricacies of the problem tempt one to predict
that a final solution will be achieved in the laboratories of the biochemist. His enzymes may have more
omnipotence of function than the surgeon's areas have
omnipresence of compartmented pathology. On the
other hand, at our present level of comprehension of
neurophysiology, there remain many unrecognized
possibilities, and certainly many surprises for our present dogma. Accordingly, any and all data obtained
by surgical investigators are welcome. What remains
obvious is that the surgery of Parkinson's disease is
not for the casually interested but must be reserved

for the serious student, endowed with special skills and opportunities for physiologic interpretation and capable of rigorous follow-up analysis of results.

REFERENCES

Aring, C. D., and Fulton, J. F.: Relation of cerebrum to cerebellum, Arch. Neurol. & Psychiat. 35:439, 1936.

Browder, J.: Section of the fibers of the anterior limb of the internal capsule in Parkinsonism, Am. J. Surg. 75:264, 1948.

Bucy, P. C.: On cortical extirpation in the treatment of involuntary movements, A. Res. Nerv. & Ment. Dis., Proc. 21:551, 1942.

Bucy, P. C., and Case, T. J.: Tremor: physiological mechanism and abolition by surgical means, Arch. Neurol. & Psychiat. 41:721, 1939.

Cooper, I.: Effects of ligation of the anterior choroidal artery on involuntary movements, Tr. Am. Neurol. A., vol. 78 (In press).

Delmas-Marsalet, P., and Bogaert, von, L.: Sur un cas de myoclonus rythmiques continués, Rev. neurol. 64:728, 1935.

Ebin, J.: Combined lateral and ventral pyramidotomy in treatment of paralysis agitans, Arch. Neurol. & Psychiat. 62:27, 1949.

Foerster, O., and Gagel, O.: Die Vorderseiten strangdurchschneidung beim menschen, Ztschr. d. ges. Neurol. u. Psychiat. 138:1, 1932.

Gardener, W. J.: Surgical aspects of Parkinson's syndrome, Postgrad. Med. 5:107, 1949.

Gowers, W. R.: In Diseases of the Nervous System, ed. 2, vol. 2, p. 657, Philadelphia, Blakiston, 1903.

Klemme, R. M.: Surgical treatment of dystonia, Res. Publ., A. Nerv. & Ment. Dis. 21:596, 1942.

Meyers, Russell: The present status of surgical procedures directed against the extrapyramidal diseases, New York J. Med., vol. 42, March 15, 1942.

Oldberg, E.: Arch. Neurol. & Psychiat. 39:272, 1938.

Oliver, L. C.: Surgery in Parkinson's disease, Lancet **256**: 910, 1949.

Parkinson: An Essay on the Shaking Palsy, London, Sherwood, Neely & Jones, 1817.

Pollock, L. J., and Davis, L.: Muscle tone in Parkinsonian states, Arch. Neurol. & Psychiat. **23**:303, 1930.

Putnam, T. J.: Results of treatment of athetosis by section of extrapyramidal tracts in the spinal cord, Arch. Neurol. & Psychiat. **39**:258, 1938.

———: Treatment of unilateral paralysis agitans by section of the lateral pyramidal tract, Arch. Neurol. & Psychiat. **44**:950, 1940.

Putnam, T. J., and Herz, E.: Results of spinal pyramidotomy in the treatment of the Parkinsonian syndrome, Arch. Neurol. & Psychiat. **63**:357, 1950.

Puusepp, L.: Chirurgische Neuropathologie Dorpat, vol. 1, p. 416, Krüger, 1932.

———: Cordotomia posterior lateralis on account of trembling and hypertonia of the muscles in the hand, Folia neuropath. eston. **10**:62, 1930.

Rizzatti, E., and Moreno, G.: Cordotomia laterale ipertonie extrapiramidale postencephalische, Schizofrenie **5**:117, 1936.

Sachs, E.: Discussion of paper by Bucy, Tr. Am. Neurol. A. **68**:80, 1942.

Walker, A. E.: Cerebral pedunculotomy for relief of involuntary movements, Acta psychiat. et neurol. **24**:723, 1949.

White, J. C.: Presentation of patient whose parkinsonian tremor had been relieved by section of the lateral segment of the cerebral peduncle, Meet. Soc. Neurol. Surgeons, Chicago, March, 1950.

INDEX

146   Index